First Edition

Copyright © May 2021 • Life & Science Publishing

1-800-336-6308 • www.mylsp.com

ISBN 978-1-953099-06-8

Printed in the USA

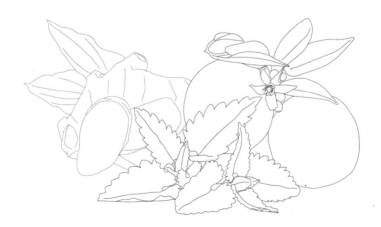

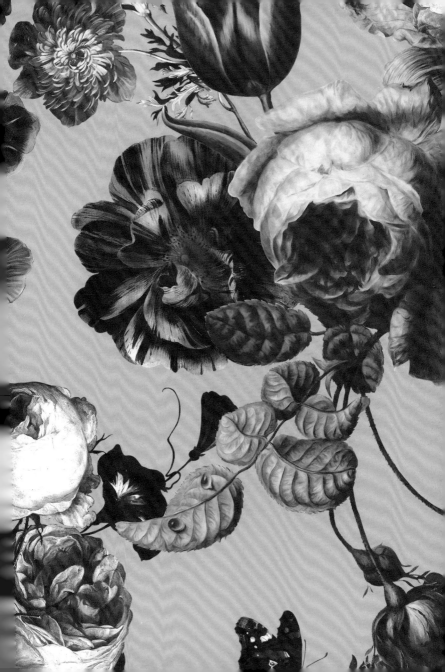

THE HEALTH + WELLNESS MANIFESTO

HEALTH AND WELLNESS ARE SIMPLE, BUT NOT EASY.

They are something we all want. The problem is that they take work -- mental, spiritual, and physical work.

WE BELIEVE THAT WORKING HARD FOR SOMETHING YOU CARE ABOUT IS CALLED "PASSION" NOT "STRESS."

Health and wellness are more than a meal plan and a gym schedule.

They are the mind, body, and soul's pursuit of joy.

WHAT OTHERS THINK ABOUT OUR CHOICE IS NOT OUR CONCERN. OUR BODIES AREN'T UP FOR DEBATE.

Our decisions don't need outside commentary.

APPROVAL ISN'T REQUIRED FOR JOY.

The way we spend our time, money, and energy should be authentic to us and the kind of life we are called to live.

JUST BECAUSE IT'S POPULAR DOESN'T MEAN IT'S GOOD FOR US.

Question everything. Do your own research. Don't take "their" word for it. Never shut up about it.

Our bodies are fearfully and wonderfully made.

We believe that the best health products aren't created in a lab -- they're made in the natural and rich soils of this amazing planet called earth.

WE ARE FEARLESS IN OUR PURSUIT OF TRUTH.

There's nothing we won't do to protect our own and our dreams for the future. There's nothing we can't do when we set our hearts and minds on a goal.

HERE'S TO US!

The wellness warriors, the healer feelers, the health nuts, the tree huggers, the essential oil freaks!

AND HERE'S TO THOSE WHO DON'T KNOW US YET -- THEY'RE ABOUT TO!

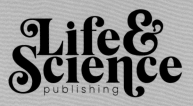

Life&Science
publishing

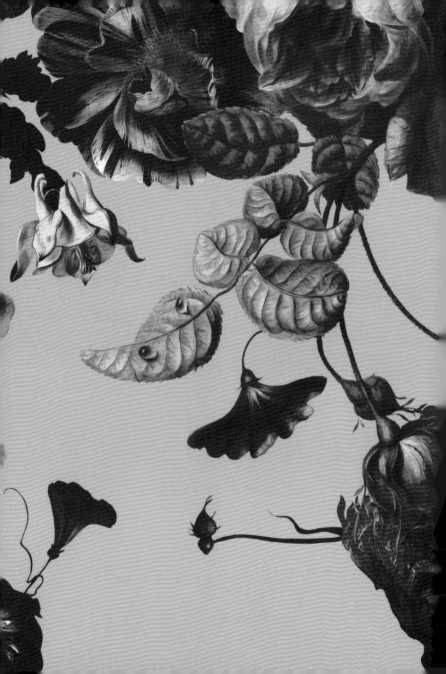

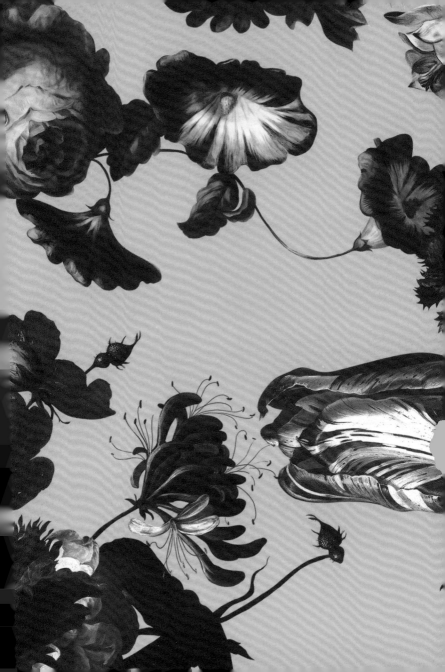

INTRODUCTION

You're our person if you're reading this right now. Holding this book in your hands means that you like the best information without taking too long to consume it. We get it, and we've got you covered on the pages of this quick reference.

Using essential oils isn't hard. Although they are mighty and versatile, it doesn't take long to understand. Many times there's a stigma attached to new or holistic things that over complicates the process. This tool will make it simple for you to grasp what's been laid out on these pages, whether you're new to this, or not.

The truth of it all is that you could use any oil, any Young Living product and it would do your body good in one way or a million.

Fast access to applicable information is the best formula for those that lead busy lives. So let's get you to that point. Let your eyes do the reading so that your hands can do the applying. Enjoy your quick dive into the deep goodness found on these pages, found in essential oils and the products made with them.

> Pro Tip: Drop this book in your bag or leave it on the counter so that you can look up that answer you're searching for, when doing your daily things at home or while on the go.

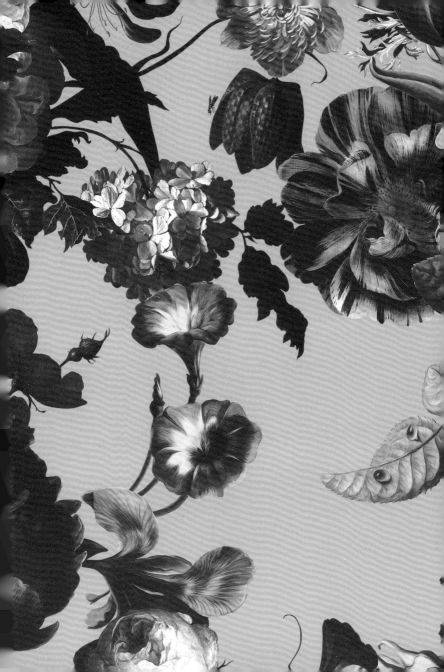

THE RIGHT KIND OF OILS

INTRODUCTION TO ESSENTIAL OILS

Let's start off with what we mean when we say "essential oils." Essential oils, known as nature's living energy, are the natural, aromatic volatile liquids found in shrubs, flowers, trees, roots, bushes, and seeds. The constituents in essential oils defend plants against insects, environmental conditions, and disease. They are also vital for a plant to grow, live, evolve, and adapt to its surroundings. Essential oils are extracted from aromatic plant sources via steam distillation, and are highly concentrated and far more potent than dry herbs.

They are not the fatty oils that we use in cooking, although many of those are great as carrier oils. They can dilute essential oils to make them less "hot" or strong on your body.

NATURALLY THERAPEUTIC™ OILS

While essential oils often have a pleasant aroma, their chemical makeup is complex and their benefits vast—which makes them much more than something that simply smells good. Mother Nature has provided a wide range of plants and essential oils. There are almost unlimited numbers of unique natural chemicals in the flowers, trees, shrubs, herbs, spices, fruits, roots, stems, leaves, and bark on this wonderful planet we call earth.

A single oil can have over 300 different natural chemical constituents. There are countless combinations. These cannot truly be synthesized in a laboratory. Even if they could, it's nearly impossible to create the same combination that Mother Nature provides. The right oils have the right constituents in the right combination to give our bodies Naturally Therapeutic™ results. Naturally Therapeutic™ oils contain the *right* extraction from the *right* plant grown under the *right* conditions.

Anyone can make an essential oil that smells good, but only the world leader can deliver proven health results. Young Living's extensive experience farming, distilling, and sourcing essential oils guarantees each Young Living oil contains the optimal level of beneficial plant properties. Oils that work — that's at the core of what it means to be Naturally Therapeutic™.

HISTORICAL USE OF ESSENTIAL OILS

Essential oils can be considered humankind's first medicine and have been used around the world for centuries. Essential oils and other aromatics have been used in religious rituals, in clearing emotional challenges, in helping support the body's natural systems, and in providing a natural alternative to other physical and spiritual needs.

Research dates the use of essential oils back to 4500 B.C. Ancient Egyptians were the first to discover the potential of aromatic compounds, and records demonstrate that oils and aromatics were used for treating illness as well as performing rituals and religious ceremonies in temples and pyramids.

According to ancient Egyptian hieroglyphics and Chinese manuscripts, priests and physicians used oils thousand of years before the time of Christ. References to oils in the Bible include some precious oils like Frankincense, Myrrh, Rosemary, Cassia, and Cinnamon.

Historically, essential oils have played a prominent role in everyday life. With more than 200 references to aromatics, incense, and ointments throughout the Bible, essential oils have played a strong role in anointing and administering to those in need. Today, essential oils are used for aromatherapy, massage therapy, emotional health, personal care, nutritional supplements, household solutions, and much more.

Young Living Essential Oils, LC the leading provider of essential oils, offers more than 300 essential oil singles and blends. All of Young Living essential oils meet the Seed to Seal® standard. This means that every essential oil Young Living distills or sources has the optimal naturally-occurring blend of constituents to maximize the desired health effects. Only Young Living's Naturally Therapeutic™ essential oils should be used for the primary methods of application, which include inhalation and topical application.

DISTILLATION OF ESSENTIAL OILS

The reintroduction of essential oils into modern medicine first began during the late 19th and early 20th centuries. Since that time essential oils have been used for physical and spiritual cleansing, enhancing spirituality, balancing mood, and dispelling negative emotions.

The key to producing a quality essential oil is to preserve the delicate compounds of the aromatic plant through expert distillation. The proper process of steam distillation—passing steam through the plant material and condensing the steam to separate the oil from the plant—is strictly adhered to with all of Young Living's essential oils.

Proper temperature must be maintained throughout the distillation process. Pressure, length of time, equipment, and batch size are strictly monitored. This ensures that the naturally-occurring compounds contained in each essential oil product are of the highest and most consistent bioactive levels.

(Please refer back to this information carefully. All directions throughout this booklet will reference these instructions.)

APPLICATION METHODS

TOPICAL

This is one of the most effective ways to use essential oils. You can simply place drops of oils directly onto the desired location of the body, or pour drops on your hands and fingers, and then gently rub them over the desired area. You may also use roll-on bottles as a convenient way to apply the oil directly on your skin.

- Neat: Apply undiluted as directed to affected area.
- Dilute 50/50: Add 1 part essential oil(s) to
  1 part V-6™ Vegetable Oil Complex.
- Dilute 20/80: Add 1 part essential oil(s) to
  4 parts V-6™ Vegetable Oil Complex.
- Vita Flex: Apply 1-3 drops directly on the Vita Flex points on the hands or feet,
  neat or diluted, as directed.
- Compress-Warm: Dilute 1 part essential oil(s) with 4 parts V-6™
  Vegetable Oil Complex and apply 8-10 drops on affected area.
  Cover with a warm, moist hand towel. Then cover the moist towel with
  a dry towel for 10-15 minutes.
- Compress-Cold: A cool, moist hand towel may also be used to
  create a cold compress in the same manner.
- Body Massage: Essential oils are typically combined with a carrier oil
  when used in massage. The diluted oil is spread over the desired
  location and then is massaged in with the hands. The oils enhance the
  power of the massage with their own unique properties.
- Baths: Essential oils are often added to baths directly or combined with
  bath salts to more easily dissolve in the bath water. The oils are drawn
  into the skin from the surrounding bath water.

INTERNALLY (See Vitality™ oils)

- Young Living's Vitality™ line is labeled for proper internal consumption.
- Gargle: Add essential oil to purified water; shake or mix vigorously.
  Gargle for 30 seconds.
- Tongue: Let 1 drop of the essential oil or blend fall from the bottle
  onto the tongue, or apply with fingertip for 1 minute, then swallow.
- Sublingual: Allow 1 drop of the oil or blend to fall under the tongue.
  Hold it there for 1-2 minutes before swallowing.
- Add 1-2 drops to a glass of pure, clean water.
- Add 1-2 drops to a vegetable capsule and swallow with 8 ounces of pure, clean water.
- Add 1-2 drops to 1 ounce of NingXia Red®.

AROMATICALLY

- Diffuse: Add several drops to an ultrasonic (cold-air) diffuser.
- Add several drops to a water-based atomizer and spray the fine mist into the air.
- Inhale Directly: Put 2-3 drops of an essential oil in the palm of one hand, rub palms together, cup hands over nose and mouth and breathe slowly. Be careful not to touch the skin near your eyes or get any oils in your eyes. If this should happen, rinse with V-6™ Vegetable Oil Complex. Do NOT rinse with water, as that will cause even more burning.

VITA FLEX

Vita Flex means "vitality through the reflexes" and is an easy way to apply essential oils through the hands and bottoms of the feet. It is a very important technique that can facilitate the relief of pain and suffering quickly, as well as improve physical and emotional well-being.

It helps identify different structural and health needs of the body and, together with the Raindrop Technique, increases the opportunity for healing and rejuvenation. Vita Flex is a specialized form of hand and foot massage that is exceptionally effective in delivering the benefits of essential oils throughout the body.
It is said to have originated in Tibet thousands of years ago and was perfected in the 1960s by Stanley Burroughs long before acupuncture was popular in Western medicine.

Vita Flex is based on a complete network of reflex points that stimulate all the internal body systems. When the fingertips connect to specific reflex points with essential oils using the special Vita Flex application, an electrical charge is released that sends energy through the neuroelectric pathways.

More than 1,500 Vita Flex points are located throughout the body in comparison to only 365 acupuncture points used in reflexology. Vita Flex is similar to but different from reflexology. As it is used today, reflexology has a tendency to ground out the electrical charge from constant compression and rotation pressure, which causes cell separation and loss of oxygen to subdermal tissues, causing further injury.

In contrast to the steady stimulation of reflexology, Vita Flex uses a rolling and releasing motion that involves placing the fingers flat on the skin, rolling up onto the fingertips, and continuing over onto the fingernails, using medium pressure, and then sliding the hand forward about $\frac{1}{2}$ inch, continually repeating this rolling and releasing technique until the specific Vita Flex area is covered. This rolling motion is repeated over the area three times.

For the areas of the body affected by the Vita Flex points, see the diagrams at the back of this booklet. For more detailed information on Vita Flex, see the *Essential Oils Complete Home Reference* or the *Essential Oils On The Go Field Reference*.

RAINDROP® TECHNIQUE

Most people would agree that massage is soothing, relaxing, and pleasurable. But Raindrop Technique is unquestionably far superior as it combines essential oils with special massage techniques to add greater therapeutic benefits to a pleasurable massage. The Raindrop Technique was developed to support health and wellness by applying oils directly to the spine in order to more quickly, directly, and deeply reach the central nervous system and energy points of the body.

In the case of Raindrop Technique, the use of certain undiluted essential oils typically causes minor reddening and "heat" in the tissues. Normally, this is perfectly safe and not something to be overly concerned about. Individuals who have fair skin such as blondes and redheads or those persons whose systems are toxic are more susceptible to this temporary irritation.

If the irritation or heat becomes excessive, it can be remedied within a minute or two by immediately applying several drops of V-6™ Vegetable Oil Complex or a pure, high-quality vegetable oil like jojoba, almond, avocado, olive, or coconut oil on the affected area. This effectively dilutes the oils and the warming effect.

RAINDROP TECHNIQUE AND ESSENTIAL OILS

Raindrop Technique is one of the safest, most noninvasive regimens available for spinal health. It is also an invaluable method for promoting healing from within using topically applied essential oils.

Single Oils

- **Oregano**: Awakens receptors, kills pathogens, and helps digest toxic substances on the receptor sites
- **Thyme**: Kills pathogens and digests waste and toxic substances on the receptor sites
- **Basil**: Releases muscle tension
- **Cypress**: Improves circulation and nourishes the pituitary gland
- **Wintergreen**: Reduces pain
- **Marjoram**: Strengthens muscles
- **Peppermint**: Promotes greater oil penetration

Essential Oil Blends

- **Valor®**: Structural balancing and alignment
- **Aroma Siez™:** Muscle relaxation and pain reduction
- **White Angelica™:** Protection for adversarial energies

Simple Explanation

The oils are dispensed like drops of rain from a height of about 6 inches above the back. Starting from the low back, the oils are feathered with the back of the fingers up along the vertebrae, out over the back muscles, and over the shoulders to the neck. Although the entire technique takes from 30-45 minutes to complete, the oils continue to work for several days as the healing and realignment processes take place.

Many recipients feel the benefits of the oils for several days afterward, as they recognize that the pain has decreased or is completely gone, there is no fever, they have more mobility, and they have an overall feeling of peace and a renewed zest for life.

The technique is very detailed and takes practice, but anyone can learn to do it. Here are the 12 summarized steps of the Raindrop Technique:

Step 1: Balance energy. Apply **Valor**® on the soles of the feet. If a second person is assisting, then that person can put the oils on the shoulders.

Step 2: Vita Flex Technique. Work the same Raindrop Technique oils into the spinal reflex areas of the feet. Vita Flex facilitates quick absorption of the oils through the bottoms of the feet and prepares the body for Raindrop on the back. It is also highly relaxing.

Step 3: The 5-step Feathering Technique. Use with each of the oils as they are applied on the back, starting at the base of the spine and working upward to stimulate the cell receptors and activate energy centers along the spine, as well as to distribute the oil drops over the back for rapid penetration.

Step 4: Feather 3-5 drops of **Oregano** from the spine outward.

Step 5: Feather 3-5 drops of **Thyme** from the spine outward.

Step 6: Stretch and release. Feather 4-6 drops of **Basil** along both sides of the spine and feather out and upward. Then take hold of the feet and gently pull to stretch the spine, releasing tension from the vertebra, back muscles, and tissue.

Step 7: Finger Straddle Massage. Apply 5-8 drops of **Cypress** on the spine and feather; then perform the Spinal Finger Straddle.

Step 8: Vita Flex Thumb Roll. Apply 5-8 drops of **Wintergreen** on the spine and feather; then perform the Vita Flex Thumb Roll.

Step 9: Circular Hand Massage. Apply 8-10 drops of **Marjoram** on the back and feather; then perform the Circular Hand Massage.

Step 10: Palm Slide. Apply 8-10 drops of **Aroma Siez™** over the entire back and feather; then perform the Palm Slide.

Step 11: Feather 3-5 drops of **Peppermint** on the spine.

Step 12: Feather 8-10 drops of **Valor**® over the back. Have the recipient finish by applying 1-2 drops of White Angelica™ on their shoulders, neck, and thymus.

For more detailed information on Raindrop Technique, see the *Essential Oils Complete Home Reference* or the *Essential Oils On The Go Field Guide*.

A Bottle Full of Raindrops
This blend is perfect to have on hand when you can't do a full Raindrop session. In a 10-ml stainless steel roller bottle, combine:

- 25 drops Valor®
- 10 drops Oregano*
- 5 drops Thyme
- 5 drops Basil
- 5 drops Cypress
- 5 drops Wintergreen*
- 5 drops Marjoram
- 5 drops Peppermint*
- 5 drops Aroma Siez
- 5 drops White Angelica

* Because these are "hot" oils, applying the blend directly to your skin may be irritating to those who are sensitive. You may want to dilute the blend by adding 1 teaspoon of V-6™ Vegetable Oil Complex to the bottle.

Apply the roller all along the spine and Vita Flex points of the feet. You can also use the Vita Flex points of the hands or roll along the backs of the ears for added effect.

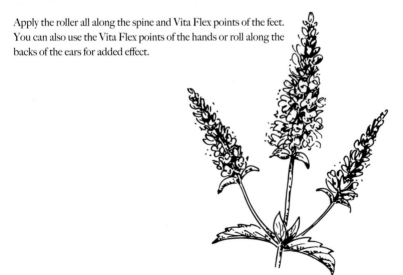

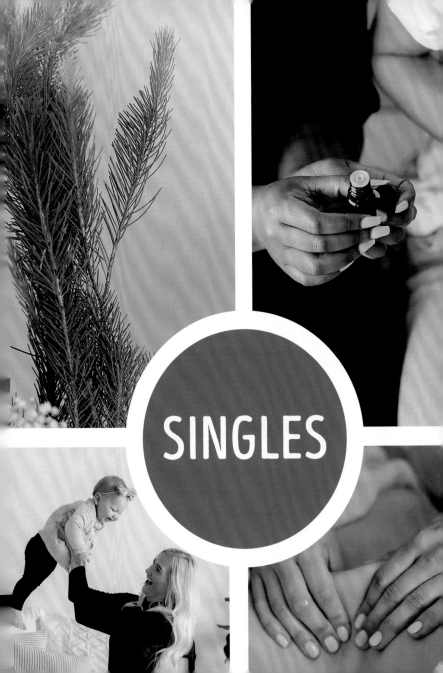

SINGLES

The oils listed within these pages are not a complete list of every oil you can use. For a complete list of oils and their possible uses, please reference the *Essential Oils Complete Home Reference* or the *Essential Oils On The Go Field Reference*.

COMMONLY USED SINGLE OILS

Experience singular notes of pure bliss. These powerful essential oils bring out the very best in you, each and every day.

Angelica (angelica archangelica)
Soothing qualities, **relax nerves and muscles**, calms anxiety, restores happy memories, brings peaceful sleep, digestive support

Balsam Fir, Idaho (abies balsamea)
Emotional balance, **muscular aches and pains**, soothes and rejuvenates body and mind

Basil (ocimum basilicum)
Mental clarity, alertness, balancing, can refresh the mind, restores mental alertness, may sharpen sense of smell, useful for fatigued or aching muscles

Bergamot (citrus bergamia)
Confidence, calming, female hormonal support, fresh sweet citrus scent, enhance mood, used for oily and troubled skin

Black Pepper (piper nigrum)
Energizing, endurance, **comforting and energizing**, used topically for soothing muscle discomfort, enhance flavor of foods

Blue Cypress (callitris intratropica)
Supports body's natural response to **irritation and injury**, aids normal breathing

Blue Tansy (tanacetum annum)
Relaxation, sweet herbaceous aroma

Cardamom (elettaria cardamomum)
Protects the stomach, invigorates the mind, alleviates mental fatigue

Carrot Seed (daucus carota)
Digestive support, joint support, **supports healthy skin**

Cedarwood (cedrus atlantica)
Balancing, relaxing, mental focus, useful for oily skin, soothing during massage

Celery Seed (apium graveolens)
Liver support, digestive support, physical discomfort

Cinnamon Bark (cinnamomum verum)
Immune system support, **promote healthy cardiovascular and immune function,** acts as
an antiseptic, dilute and use for massage

Cistus (cistus ladanifer)
Relaxing and elevating, **calming, uplifting,** helpful for meditating and counseling

Citronella (cymbopogon nardus)
Respiratory support, **insect repellent,** relaxing, can delay food spoilage due to fungus

Clary Sage (salvia sclarea)
Stress relief, **female hormonal support,** relaxing, supports normal healthy attitude during
PMS

Clove (syzygium aromaticum)
Antioxidant support, digestive support, physical discomfort, stimulating and revitalizing

Copaiba (copaifera reticulata)
Physical discomfort, aids digestion, and **supports body's natural response to injury or
irritation**

Coriander (coriandrum sativum)
Pancreatic support, digestive support, soothing and calming properties, **supports healthy
digestive and circulatory system functions**

Cypress (cupressus sempervirens)
Grounding, **restores feelings of security and stability,** beneficial for oily or troubled skin

Dill (anethum graveolens)
Flavorant, calming, digestive support, **balancing, stimulating, and revitalizing**

Dorado Azul
Supports the respiratory tract, balances hormones, soothes skin, invigorates the senses

Elemi (canarium luzonicum)
Grounding, traditionally used for skin, **reduce look of fine lines and wrinkles**, soothing muscles

Eucalyptus Blue
Supports respiratory system, has a cooling and invigorating effect

Eucalyptus Globulus (eucalyptus globulus)
Key ingredient in many mouth rinses, **applied topically in respiratory system**, soothe muscles after exercise

Eucalyptus Radiata (eucalyptus radiata)
Purifying, cleansing, relatively gentle and non-irritating, suitable for topical use

Fennel (foeniculum vulgare)
Women's health, digestive support, **stimulating to circulatory, glandular, respiratory and digestive systems**, support during menstrual cycle

Frankincense (boswellia carteri)
Immune support, skin health, spiritual grounding, stimulating and elevating to the mind, help focus the mind, overcome stress and despair

Galbanum (ferula gummosa)
Spiritual grounding, **supports systems** including immune, digestive, respiratory, and circulatory

Geranium (pelargonium graveolens)
Respiratory support, liver support, women's health, excellent for the skin, helps release negative memories, supports circulatory and nervous systems

German Chamomile (matricaria recutita)
Liver and gallbladder support, **relaxing**, supports natural response to irritation and injury

Ginger (zingiber officinale)
Muscle tension, **digestive support**, stamina

Goldenrod (solidago canadensis)
Libido, circulatory support, **supports urinary tract, liver function**

Grapefruit (citrus paradisi)
Energizing and uplifting, nourishes the skin

Helichrysum (helichrysum italicum)
Circulatory support, muscle tension, restorative properties, supports nervous system, skin, liver

Hinoki (chamaecyparis obtusa)
Spiritual awareness, energizes and uplifts the mind, calming and relaxing during agitation

Hong Kuai (chamaecyparis formosensis)
Supports deep sense of relaxation, spiritual awareness, abundant aromatic nature

Hyssop (hyssopus officinalis)
Slightly sweet, purifying

Idaho Blue Spruce
Muscle tension, emotional release

Idaho Tansy (tanacetum vulgare)
Stimulates positive attitude and general feeling of well-being, soothing to the skin

Jasmine (jasminum officinale)
Relaxes, soothes, uplifts and enhances self-confidence, used to balance feminine energy

Juniper (Juniperus osteosperma and scopulorum)
Cleansing effect on the mind, spirit and body, detoxifier and cleanser, beneficial to the skin

Laurus Nobilis (laurus nobilis)
Respiratory support, grounding, calming

Lavender (lavandula angustifolia)
Skin irritations, balancing, relaxing, soothing and refreshing, good for relaxing and winding down before bedtime, boosts stamina

Ledum (ledum groenlandicum)
Cleansing, provides well-being, believed to harmonize and balance the body's daily needs

Lemon (citrus limon)
Energizing, circulatory support, cleansing, beneficial to the skin, enhance flavor of foods, supports nervous and sympathetic systems

Lemon Myrtle (backhousia citriodora)
Mental clarity, **immune support**, purifying, boosts natural defenses, can act as cleansing agent to purify household surfaces

Lemongrass (cymbopogon flexuosus)
Purifying, digestive support, rejuvenating, improves mental clarity, supports circulatory system

Lime (citrus latifolia)
Invigorating and stimulating effect, may help mental clarity and **encourage creativity**, supports healthy immune system

Marjoram (origanum majorana)
Muscle tension, calming, relaxing, occasional simple nervous tension

Melaleuca Quinquenervia (niaouli)
Supports **skin health**

Melissa (melissa officinalis)
Strengthening and revitalizing, soothing and calming, may benefit the skin, **supports immune system**

Mountain Savory (satureja montana)
General tonic for the body, **provides support for the immune, nervous, and circulatory systems**

Myrrh (commipihora myrrha)
Spiritual awareness, skin health, **antioxidant support**, revitalizing and uplifting, widely used in oral hygiene products

Myrtle (Myrtus communis)
Respiratory support, thyroid support, emotional balance, **supportive system for skin and hair**

Neroli (citrus aurantium)
Mental clarity, emotional balance, believed to have **healing properties**

Nutmeg (myristica fragrans)
Energizing, helps boost energy, **supports nervous and endocrine systems**

Ocotea (ocotea quixos)
Purifying, digestive support, satiety, **helps aid body's natural response to irritation and injury**

Orange (citrus sinensis)
Cellular support, **uplifting, emotional balance,** calming influence on the body, aids in maintaining normal cellular regeneration

Oregano (origanum vulgare)
Purifying, **contains strong immune enhancing and antioxidant properties,** supports respiratory system

Palmarosa (cymbopogon martini)
Cellular support, **skin health,** balancing

Palo Santo (bursera graveolens)
Spiritual grounding, emotional balance, used to purify and cleanse the spirit of negative energies

Patchouli (pogostemon cablin)
Skin health, **emotional release,** anti-nausea support, general health support, releases negative emotions

Peppermint (mentha piperita)
Energizing, digestive support, may improve taste and smell when inhaled, may help improve concentration and mental sharpness

Petitgrain (citrus sinensis)
Skin health, emotional balance, **nervous system support,** beneficial for skin and hair health

Pine (pinus sylvestris)
Respiratory support, emotional balance, **soothes stressed muscles and joints** when used in massage

Ravintsara (cinnamomum camphora)
Purifying, meditation, **similar to eucalyptus but softer, spicy**

Roman Chamomile (chamaemelum nobile)
Skin health, relaxing, muscle tension, **gentle effects especially valuable for restless children,** beneficial when added to massage oil

Rose (rosa damascena)
Skin health, emotional release, energy balance, simulating and uplifting properties

Rosemary (rosmarinus officinalis CT cineol)
Mental clarity, liver support, may help restore mental alertness when experiencing fatigue

Royal Hawaiian Sandalwood (santalum paniculatum)
Uplifting, relaxing, valued in **skin care**, moisturizing and normalizing properties

Sacred Frankincense™ (boswellia sacra)
Ideal for those wishing to take **their spiritual journey and meditation** experiences to a higher level

Sage (salvia officinalis)
Mental balance, **skin health, women's health**, supports respiratory, reproductive, and nervous systems

Spearmint (nentha spicata)
Emotional release, **digestive support**, respiratory health, leads to sense of balance and well-being

Spikenard (nardostachys jatamansi)
Relaxing, **soothing for the skin**

Lavender (lavandula angustifolia)
Skin irritations, balancing, relaxing, **soothes and cleanses minor cuts, bruises and skin irritations**

Tangerine (citrus reticulata)
Antioxidant support, digestive support, satiety, **uplifts the spirit** and brings sense of security

Tarragon (artemisia dracunculus)
Digestive support, adds special touch when used as a spice in recipes

Tea Tree (Melaleuca alternifolia)
Cleansing, supports immune system and **benefits the skin**

Thyme (thymus vulgaris)
Immune support, purifying, cleansing, **supports immune, respiratory, digestive, nervous, and other body systems**

Tsuga (tsuga canadensis)
Spiritual balance, used to make poultices, for wounds, **skin cleansing**

Valerian (valeriana officinalis)
Calming, sleep support, emotional balance, believed to have relaxing properties, calming and restorative effects on nervous system

Vetiver (vetiveria zizanoides)
Emotional grounding, sleep support, relaxing, supports **coping with stress** and recovering from emotional trauma and shock

Wintergreen (gaultheria procumbens)
Flavors numerous products, beneficial in massage and soothing head tension and muscles after exercising, **pain in bones and joints**

Xiang Mao (cymbopogon citratus)
Spiritual awareness, **calming, relaxing, and cleansing**

Ylang Ylang (cananga odorata)
Circulatory support, emotional balance

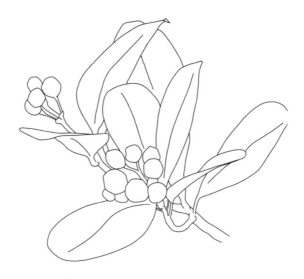

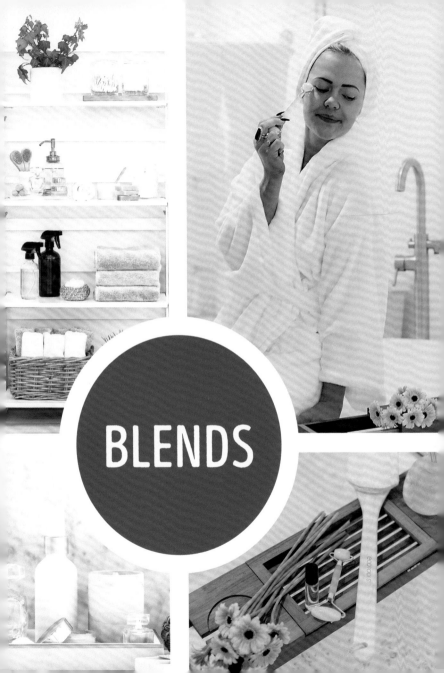

BLENDS

COMMONLY USED BLENDS

Transform your day and awaken your senses with formulated essential oil blends designed to meet your daily needs.

Abundance™
Emotional support, energizing, **attracts prosperity.**
Abundance™ opens us to a wealth of possibilities

Acceptance™
Self-worth, stimulates the mind, helps **overcome procrastination and denial**

Aroma Life™
Combines Ylang Ylang with known powerhouses **Cypress, Helichrysum, and Marjoram**

Aroma Siez™
Well suited for use after exercise, combined with massage oil, provides soothing comfort for head, neck, and tired feet, **helps muscle release**

AromaEase™
Soothes occasional stress, helps **support healthy energy flow and vitality**

Australian Blue™
Uplifts and inspires the mind and heart, calming and stabilizing

Awaken™
Helps **awaken potential,** supports making necessary changes to manifest dreams and goals

Brain Power™
Use it to **clarify thought and develop focus**

Build Your Dream™
Includes significant oils that highlight a lifetime journey of helping individuals **discover profound and lasting transformations,** improve their health, and change lives around the world

Christmas Spirit™
Purifies and balances energy, helps tap into **happiness, joy and security** associated with the holiday season

Citrus Fresh™
Mental clarity, energizing, purifying, supports immune system, and overall health

Clarity™
Promotes mental sharpness, restores mental alertness or wakefulness when you're fatigued or drowsy

Common Sense™
Enhances rational decision making abilities, leading to increased wellness, purpose, and abundance

DiGize™
Helps support a **healthy digestive system**

Dragon Time™
Perfect choice for **women's emotions during special times and needs.** Promotes balance and normal healthy emotions

Dream Catcher™
Spiritual awareness, **enhances ability to hold onto dreams,** protects against negative dreams that may cloud vision

Egyptian Gold™
Spiritual awareness, **immune support,** enhances moments of devotion and reverence

En-R-Gee™
Helps restore mental alertness, **boosts energy**

Endoflex™
Endocrine support, female hormonal support

Envision™
Emotional release, renew focus, **stimulates creativity and resourcefulness,** encourages renewed faith in the future

Evergreen Essence™
Refreshes the senses, get back to nature by combining aromatic scents of pine, cedar, and spruce trees

Exodus II™
Cleansing, timeless blend of oils

Forgiveness™
Emotional support, emotional release, energy balance, soothing and uplifting oils that may enhance the ability to release hurtful memories and move beyond emotional barriers

GLF™
Blend of powerful oils including Helichrysum, Spearmint, and Celery Seed, **applied topically over the liver** and on Vita Flex points on the feet

Gathering™
Spiritual grounding, emotional balance, **helps overcome chaotic energy**, helps gather emotional and spiritual forces to achieve greater unity of purpose

Gentle Baby™
Calming, relaxing, designed especially for mothers and babies, helps calm emotions during pregnancy and is useful for quieting little ones, **soothing to tender skin**

Gratitude™
Spiritual grounding, emotional balance, **designed to elevate the spirit**, calm emotions, fosters grateful attitude

Grounding™
Mental clarity, stress relief, emotional balance, may aid in coping with reality in a positive way

Harmony™
Stress relief, energy balance, promotes physical and emotional well-being by bringing **harmonic balance to the energy** centers of the body

Highest Potential™
Confidence, emotional balance, **designed to increase your capacity** to achieve your highest potential, soothes, and harmonizes

Hope™
Emotional grounding, emotional strength, **designed to uplift and balance emotions**, may help to overcome severe dark thoughts

Humility™
Spiritual awareness, emotional balance, emotional strength, may bring balance to your heart and mind, promoting emotional healing

ImmuPower™
Creates a fragrant and protective haven while increasing positive energy, **supports immune system**

Inner Child™
Emotional release, emotional balance, **opens pathways to connect with the inner self** that may have been misused or abused in childhood

Inspiration™
Spiritual awareness, **calming, enhancing spirituality,** prayer, meditation, and inner awareness, creates aromatic sanctuary

Into the Future™
Confidence, decision-making, emotional release, **fosters feelings of determination,** leaving the past behind so you can move forward, enhances enjoyment of challenges

Joy™
Emotional balance, uplifting, **creates magnetic energy and brings joy to the heart,** may exude an irresistible fragrance inspiring togetherness

JuvaCleanse®
Supports normal **liver function,** balancing

JuvaFlex™
Liver support, digestive support, may also **support healthy cell function**

Lady Sclareol™
Designed as an exquisite fragrance, creating a beguiling and alluring perfume, **hormone support**

Live with Passion™
Helps revive the zest for life, **improves internal energy,** formulated specifically to help recover an optimistic attitude

Longevity™
Antioxidant support, help neutralizes free radicals and lessen the daily oxidative damage

M-Grain™
Calming, promotes sense of well-being particularly in the head and neck area, **soothes headaches**

Magnify Your Purpose™
Mental clarity, motivation, stimulates desire, focus and motivation, helps **foster positive attitude**

Melrose™
Skin health, cleansing, provides a protective barrier against skin challenges, can help dispel odors

Mister™
Emotional balance, helps promote greater inner body balance, may be soothing while stressed, **recommended for males 30 years and over**

Motivation™
Positive energy, emotional release, motivation, may help enable one to **surmount fear and procrastination,** while stimulating feelings of action and accomplishment

PanAway®
Often used for massage and soothing skin, while providing **comfort to muscles** after exercise

Peace & Calming®
Gentle fragrant blend, helps **calm tension and uplift the spirit,** promotes relaxation and a deep sense of peace

Present Time™
Empowerment, **emotional release,** may heighten the sense of being "in the moment"

Purification®
Cleansing, **used directly on skin to clean and soothe,** helps purify air when diffused

R.C.™
May be invigorating when applied to chest and throat, wonderful blend to diffuse during winter, **supports respiratory system**

Raven™
Combination of soothing oils, provides comfort when applied topically to chest and throat or when diffused, **supports respiratory system**

Release™
Emotional release and balance, stimulates sense of peace and emotional well-being, may facilitate the ability to **release anger and frustration**

Relieve It™
Deeply relaxing, **soothing and comforting to muscles and joints** following exercise

RutaVaLa™
Stress relieving, relaxing, helps ease tension

SARA™
Emotional release, emotional healing, relaxing, may help soothe deep emotional wounds

Sacred Mountain™
Empowerment, emotional balance, emotional strength, **promotes feelings of strength, grounding, and protection**

SclarEssence™
Female hormonal support, energy balance, women's health, calming action for an extraordinary dietary supplement

Sensation™
Romantic emotions, skin health, **extremely uplifting and refreshing**

Slique™ Essence
Weight management support, **satiety, supports healthy weight management goals,** may help with hunger and digestion

Stress Away™
Designed to **combat normal everyday stresses**, reduce mental rigidity, and restore equilibrium

Surrender™
Emotional release and balance, helps quiet troubled hearts so that negative emotions can be released, return feelings of equilibrium

The Gift™
Immune support, calming effects

Thieves®
Immune support, purifying, tested for its cleansing abilities, supports good health

Three (3) Wise Men™
Spiritual awareness, **promotes feelings of reverence**, formulated to open the subconscious

Transformation™
Emotional release, empowers you to **replace negative beliefs with uplifting thoughts,** changing your overall attitude, emotions, and behavior

Trauma Life™
Stress relief, **emotional release,** formulated to help release buried emotional trauma resulting from accidents, neglect, death, assault or abuse

White Angelica™
Spiritual awareness, energy balance, encourages feelings of protection and security to bring about sense of strength and endurance

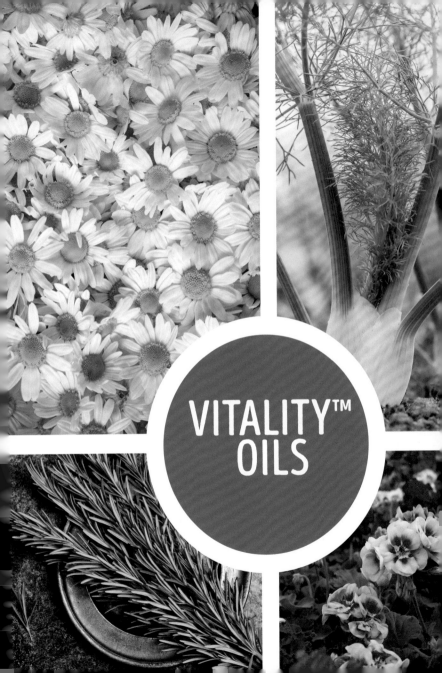

COMMONLY USED VITALITY™ OILS

Why use Vitality™ oils? Amazing flavor + additional health support! What could be better? Young Living's Vitality™ Line contains over 40 delicious, valuable dietary-grade essential oils that can be added to your favorite dishes for a pop of flavor, used as a substitute for dried or fresh ingredients, or taken in capsules for their health boosting properties.

HERB

Basil Vitality™ easily pairs with savory foods, but can also complement any meal with its sweet, slightly peppery flavor that also **aids in healthy digestion**.

- **Dressings** - Add 1-2 drops and shake to combine
- **Pastas** - Dip a toothpick and stir until desired flavor
- **Soups** - Stir in 1-2 drops
- **Marinades** - Mix in 1-2 drops
- **Sauces** - Add 1-2 drops and mix well

Carrot Seed Vitality™ offers a strong, earthy flavor that richens any dish and **helps fight inflammation in your body**.

- **Dressings** - Add 1-2 drops and shake to combine
- **Soups** - Stir in 1-2 drops
- **Marinades** - Mix in 1-2 drops
- **Sauces** - Add 1-2 drops and mix well
- **Baked Goods** - Blend 1-2 drops into batter

Celery Seed Vitality™ has a grassy and earthy flavor that can quickly bring a pleasant taste and aroma as well as **helps maintain a healthy blood pressure**.

- **Dressings** - Add 1-2 drops and shake to combine
- **Pastas** - Dip a toothpick and stir until desired flavor
- **Soups** - Stir in 1-2 drops
- **Marinades** - Mix in 1-2 drops
- **Sauces** - Add 1-2 drops and mix well

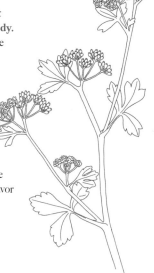

Cilantro Vitality™ adds a bright, tangy flavor that not only boosts your dish, but your **immune system too!**
- **Dressings** - Add 1-2 drops and shake to combine
- **Soups** - Stir in 1-2 drops
- **Marinades** - Mix in 1-2 drops
- **Sauces** - Add 1-2 drops and mix well
- **Dips** - Blend in 1-2 drops

Dill Vitality™ combines a fresh, grassy tone with a hint of citrus that boldens any dish it is added to and **helps maintain healthy cholesterol levels.**
- **Dressings** - Add 1-2 drops and shake to combine
- **Soups** - Stir in 1-2 drops
- **Marinades** - Mix in 1-2 drops
- **Sauces** - Add 1-2 drops and mix well
- **Dips** - Blend in 1-2 drops

Fennel Vitality™ has a distinct licorice flavor that enhances other sweet flavors and **supports a healthy heart.**
- **Dressings** - Add 1-2 drops and shake to combine
- **Marinades** - Mix in 1-2 drops
- **Hot Drinks** - Add 1 drop per 8 oz and stir
- **Sauces** - Add 1-2 drops and mix well
- **Baked Goods** - Blend 1-2 drops into batter

Steamed from elegant flowers, **German Chamomile Vitality**™ has a delicate apple taste that boosts the sweetness of flavors and helps settle your stomach and your mind.
- **Dressings** - Add 1-2 drops and shake to combine
- **Soups** - Stir in 1-2 drops
- **Hot Drinks** - Add 1 drop per 8 oz and stir
- **Sauces** - Add 1-2 drops and mix well
- **Baked Goods** - Blend 1-2 drops into batter

More commonly known as bay leaf, **Larus Nobilis Vitality**™ has soft tones of pepper and mint that add warmth and lightness to otherwise heavy dishes- all while fighting **inflammation and infection**.
- **Pastas** - Dip a toothpick and stir until desired flavor
- **Soups** - Stir in 1-2 drops
- **Marinades** - Mix in 1-2 drops
- **Hot Drinks** - Add 1 drop per 8 oz and stir
- **Sauces** - Add 1-2 drops and mix well

Lavender Vitality™ has a strong, floral taste that adds a unique and sophisticated flavor to your dishes with added **anti-inflammatory benefits**.
- **Dressings** - Add 1-2 drops and shake to combine
- **Soups** - Stir in 1-2 drops
- **Hot or Cold Drinks** - Add 1 drop per 8 oz and stir
- **Baked Goods** - Blend 1-2 drops into batter
- **Dips** - Blend in 1-2 drops

Lemongrass Vitality™ has a delicate citrus flavor that brightens and enriches dishes while simultaneously **supporting your overall wellness**.
- **Dressings** - Add 1-2 drops and shake to combine
- **Pastas** - Dip a toothpick and stir until desired flavor
- **Soups** - Stir in 1-2 drops
- **Marinades** - Mix in 1-2 drops
- **Cold Drinks** - Add 1 drop per 8 oz and stir

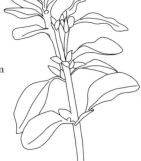

Marjoram Vitality™ **promotes healthy blood circulation** and offers a similar taste to Oregano, but with sharper hints of sweetness and warmth.
- **Pastas** - Dip a toothpick and stir until desired flavor
- **Soups** - Stir in 1-2 drops
- **Marinades** - Mix in 1-2 drops
- **Hot Drinks** - Add 1 drop per 8 oz and stir
- **Sauces** - Add 1-2 drops and mix well

The spicy, herbaceous flavor of **Mountain Savory Vitality**™ adds a strong warm flavor that is **soothing to the body.**
- **Pastas** - Dip a toothpick and stir until desired flavor
- **Soups** - Stir in 1-2 drops
- **Marinades** - Mix in 1-2 drops
- **Hot Drinks** - Add 1 drop per 8 oz and stir
- **Sauces** - Add 1-2 drops and mix well

A subtle balance between sweet and spicy, **Oregano Vitality**™ adds bold flavor to your dish with added **antibiotic benefits**.
- **Dressings** - Add 1-2 drops and shake to combine
- **Pastas** - Dip a toothpick and stir until desired flavor
- **Soups** - Stir in 1-2 drops
- **Marinades** - Mix in 1-2 drops
- **Sauces** - Add 1-2 drops and mix well

Parsley Vitality™ has a clean, peppery taste that enhances other elements in your dish as well as **aids in digestion**.
- **Dressings** - Add 1-2 drops and shake to combine
- **Pastas** - Dip a toothpick and stir until desired flavor
- **Soups** - Stir in 1-2 drops
- **Sauces** - Add 1-2 drops and mix well
- **Dips** - Blend in 1-2 drops

Peppermint Vitality™ offers a bright and cool flavor with added benefits of **digestive support and energy**.
- **Dressings** - Add 1-2 drops and shake to combine
- **Soups** - Stir in 1-2 drops
- **Hot or Cold Drinks** - Add 1 drop per 8 oz and stir
- **Baked Goods** - Blend 1-2 drops into batter
- **Dips** - Blend in 1-2 drops

Rosemary Vitality™ has a diverse flavor profile encompassing minty, woody, and sweet tones, all combined for amazing flavor and **anti-inflammatory properties**.
- **Pastas** - Dip a toothpick and stir until desired flavor
- **Soups** - Stir in 1-2 drops
- **Marinades** - Mix in 1-2 drops
- **Sauces** - Add 1-2 drops and mix well
- **Dips** - Blend in 1-2 drops

Sage Vitality™ is known for its warm, earthy flavor that enriches any dish it is added to, while **helping your body refresh and eliminate toxins.**
- **Dressings** - Add 1-2 drops and shake to combine
- **Soups** - Stir in 1-2 drops
- **Marinades** - Mix in 1-2 drops
- **Sauces** - Add 1-2 drops and mix well
- **Baked Goods** - Blend 1-2 drops into batter

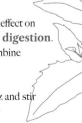

Sweet yet spicy, **Spearmint Vitality**™ has a cooling effect on foods that is both pleasing to taste and **beneficial for digestion**.
- **Dressings** - Add 1-2 drops and shake to combine
- **Soups** - Stir in 1-2 drops
- **Marinades** - Mix in 1-2 drops
- **Hot or Cold Drinks** - Add 1 drop per 8 oz and stir
- **Baked Goods** - Blend 1-2 drops into batter

Tarragon Vitality™ boosts blood circulation and offers a unique combination of sweetness and bitterness with a hint of licorice that add richness and depth to your favorite foods.

- **Dressings** - Add 1-2 drops and shake to combine
- **Soups** - Stir in 1-2 drops
- **Marinades** - Mix in 1-2 drops
- **Hot Drinks** - Add 1 drop per 8 oz and stir
- **Sauces** - Add 1-2 drops and mix well

Thyme Vitality™ has a classic flavor that perfectly combines herbaceous tones with floral notes, while **supporting a healthy immune system**.

- **Dressings** - Add 1-2 drops and shake to combine
- **Pastas** - Dip a toothpick and stir until desired flavor
- **Soups** - Stir in 1-2 drops
- **Marinades** - Mix in 1-2 drops
- **Sauces** - Add 1-2 drops and mix well

SPICE

Black Pepper Vitality™ has a strong, earthy flavor that enhances the depth of your dish and **provides great antioxidant properties**.

- **Dressings** - Add 1-2 drops and shake to combine
- **Soups** - Stir in 1-2 drops
- **Marinades** - Mix in 1-2 drops
- **Sauces** - Add 1-2 drops and mix well
- **Dips** - Blend in 1-2 drops

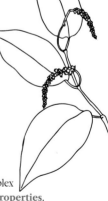

A few drops of **Caraway Vitality**™ **can help ease heartburn** while adding a unique nutty flavor to foods.

- **Dressings** - Add 1-2 drops and shake to combine
- **Soups** - Stir in 1-2 drops
- **Marinades** - Mix in 1-2 drops
- **Hot Drinks** - Add 1 drop per 8 oz and stir
- **Sauces** - Add 1-2 drops and mix well

Minty, citrusy, and earthy, **Cardamom Vitality**™ has a complex flavor that combines all your favorite flavors and **has digestive properties**.

- **Soups** - Stir in 1-2 drops
- **Hot drinks** - Add 1 drop per 8 oz and stir
- **Sauces** - Add 1-2 drops and mix well
- **Baked Goods** - Blend 1-2 drops into batter
- **Dips** - Blend in 1-2 drops

Cinnamon Bark Vitality™ essential oil has a warm, spicy flavor that is great for boosting flavors and your **immune system.**

- **Soups** - Stir in 1-2 drops
- **Hot and cold drinks** - Add 1 drop per 8 oz and stir
- **Sauces** - Add 1-2 drops and mix well
- **Baked Goods** - Blend 1-2 drops into batter
- **Dips** - Blend in 1-2 drops

Warm and spicy, **Clove Vitality**™ contains the naturally occurring constituent eugenol that doubles as a flavor enhancer and **immunity booster.**

- **Soups** - Stir in 1-2 drops
- **Marinades** - Mix in 1-2 drops
- **Hot Drinks** - Add 1 drop per 8 oz and stir
- **Sauces** - Add 1-2 drops and mix well
- **Baked Goods** - Blend 1-2 drops into batter

The flavor of **Cumin Vitality**™ combines hints of warmth and citrus that add depth to your favorite dishes while **aiding your body's ability to fight infection.**

- **Dressings** - Add 1-2 drops and shake to combine
- **Soups** - Stir in 1-2 drops
- **Marinades** - Mix in 1-2 drops
- **Sauces** - Add 1-2 drops and mix well
- **Dips** - Blend in 1-2 drops

Ginger Vitality™ has some of the most versatile uses because of its bold but blending flavor profile, as well as its **ability to fight nausea and promote healthy digestion.**

- **Dressings** - Add 1-2 drops and shake to combine
- **Marinades** - Mix in 1-2 drops
- **Hot and Cold Drinks** - Add 1 drop per 8 oz and stir
- **Sauces** - Add 1-2 drops and mix well
- **Baked Goods** - Blend 1-2 drops into batter

Nutmeg Vitality™ has a sweet yet spicy taste that compliments and enhances other flavors while **boosting cognitive function.**

- **Soups** - Stir in 1-2 drops
- **Marinades** - Mix in 1-2 drops
- **Hot and Cold Drinks** - Add 1 drop per 8 oz and stir
- **Sauces** - Add 1-2 drops and mix well
- **Baked Goods** - Blend 1-2 drops into batter

Bright and warm, **Coriander Vitality**™ enhances the flavors its paired with and **helps you maintain healthy blood sugar levels.**
- **Dressings** - Add 1-2 drops and shake to combine
- **Soups** - Stir in 1-2 drops
- **Marinades** - Mix in 1-2 drops
- **Sauces** - Add 1-2 drops and mix well
- **Dips** - Blend in 1-2 drops

CITRUS

Bergamot Vitality™ has a fresh, tart, citrus flavor that adds light to your dish and **energy to your day.**
- **Dressings** - Add 1-2 drops and shake to combine
- **Marinades** - Mix in 1-2 drops
- **Cold Drinks** - Add 1 drop per 8 oz and stir
- **Baked Goods** - Blend 1-2 drops into batter
- **Dips** - Blend in 1-2 drops

Citrus Fresh Vitality™ brings together Orange, Grapefruit, Mandarin, Tangerine, and Lemon with a splash of Spearmint to **help cleanse your body** and brighten your dishes.
- **Dressings** - Add 1-2 drops and shake to combine
- **Marinades** - Mix in 1-2 drops
- **Hot or Cold Drinks** - Add 1 drop per 8 oz and stir
- **Baked Goods** - Blend 1-2 drops into batter
- **Dips** - Blend in 1-2 drops

Tangy and tart, **Grapefruit Vitality**™ adds excitement and freshness to your favorite flavors while **helping you maintain a healthy lymphatic system and weight.**
- **Dressings** - Add 1-2 drops and shake to combine
- **Marinades** - Mix in 1-2 drops
- **Hot and Cold Drinks** - Add 1 drop per 8 oz and stir
- **Baked Goods** - Blend 1-2 drops into batter
- **Dips** - Blend in 1-2 drops

A fun lemon- lime fusion, **Jade Lemon Vitality**™ enlivens your recipes and your body with its **antioxidant properties** in every drop.
- **Dressings** - Add 1-2 drops and shake to combine
- **Marinades** - Mix in 1-2 drops
- **Hot and Cold Drinks** - Add 1 drop per 8 oz and stir
- **Baked Goods** - Blend 1-2 drops into batter
- **Dips** - Blend in 1-2 drops

Popular for its **cleansing and uplifting properties, Lemon Vitality™** is a great addition to perk up any dish.

- **Dressings** - Add 1-2 drops and shake to combine
- **Pastas** - Dip a toothpick and stir until desired flavor
- **Marinades** - Mix in 1-2 drops
- **Hot and Cold Drinks** - Add 1 drop per 8 oz and stir
- **Baked Goods** - Blend 1-2 drops into batter

Grab **Lime Vitality™** to add some zip to your dishes with its bright, crisp flavor that **boosts a healthy immune system** as well as your favorite flavors.

- **Dressings** - Add 1-2 drops and shake to combine
- **Marinades** - Mix in 1-2 drops
- **Hot or Cold Drinks** - Add 1 drop per 8 oz and stir
- **Baked Goods** - Blend 1-2 drops into batter
- **Dips** - Blend in 1-2 drops

Orange Vitality™ adds freshness and fun to everything it combines with – not to mention its amazing **cleansing and detoxing abilities.**

- **Dressings** - Add 1-2 drops and shake to combine
- **Marinades** - Mix in 1-2 drops
- **Hot and Cold Drinks** - Add 1 drop per 8 oz and stir
- **Sauces** - Add 1-2 drops and mix well
- **Baked Goods** - Blend 1-2 drops into batter

The sweetest of the citruses, **Tangerine Vitality™** adds vibrancy to dishes and your **mental state.**

- **Dressings** - Add 1-2 drops and shake to combine
- **Marinades** - Mix in 1-2 drops
- **Hot and Cold Drinks** - Add 1 drop per 8 oz and stir
- **Baked Goods** - Blend 1-2 drops into batter
- **Dips** - Blend in 1-2 drops

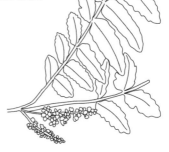

SUPPLEMENT

Copaiba Vitality™ has many benefits to the body, including **supporting cardiovascular, immune, digestive, and nervous system function.**
- **Dressings** - Add 1-2 drops and shake to combine
- **Pastas** - Dip a toothpick and stir until desired flavor
- **Soups** - Stir in 1-2 drops
- **Hot Drinks** - Add 1 drop per 8 oz and stir
- **Sauces** - Add 1-2 drops and mix well

DiGize Vitality™ combines Tarragon, Ginger, Peppermint, Juniper, Fennel, Lemongrass, Anise, and Patchouli for a unique flavor and **abundance of antioxidant benefits.**
- **Dressings** - Add 1-2 drops and shake to combine
- **Pastas** - Dip a toothpick and stir until desired flavor
- **Soups** - Stir in 1-2 drops
- **Sauces** - Add 1-2 drops and mix well
- **Dips** - Blend in 1-2 drops

EndoFlex Vitality™ features Spearmint, Sage, Geranium, Myrtle, Nutmeg, and German Chamomile – all amazing flavors, all **powerful antioxidants.**
- **Dressings** - Add 1-2 drops and shake to combine
- **Soups** - Stir in 1-2 drops
- **Marinades** - Mix in 1-2 drops
- **Hot and Cold Drinks** - Add 1 drop per 8 oz and stir
- **Sauces** - Add 1-2 drops and mix well

Frankincense Vitality™ offers a rich, diverse flavor that also **supports strong cellular function.**
- **Pastas** - Dip a toothpick and stir until desired flavor
- **Soups** - Stir in 1-2 drops
- **Marinades** - Mix in 1-2 drops
- **Hot Drinks** - Add 1 drop per 8 oz and stir
- **Baked Goods** - Blend 1-2 drops into batter

GLF Vitality™ combines some of Young Living's most popular and powerful oils to **support healthy liver and gallbladder function**.
- **Dressings** - Add 1-2 drops and shake to combine
- **Marinades** - Mix in 1-2 drops
- **Hot and Cold Drinks** - Add 1 drop per 8 oz and stir
- **Sauces** - Add 1-2 drops and mix well
- **Dips** - Blend in 1-2 drops

JuvaCleanse Vitality™ is formulated to have rich, cleansing properties that help **support digestion and a healthy immune system.**

- **Dressings** - Add 1-2 drops and shake to combine
- **Soups** - Stir in 1-2 drops
- **Marinades** - Mix in 1-2 drops
- **Hot Drinks** - Add 1 drop per 8 oz and stir
- **Sauces** - Add 1-2 drops and mix well

Part of Young Living's Golden Touch 1™ collection, **JuvaFlex Vitality**™ is known for its ability to **aid in overall, body function.**

- **Dressings** - Add 1-2 drops and shake to combine
- **Soups** - Stir in 1-2 drops
- **Marinades** - Mix in 1-2 drops
- **Hot and Cold Drinks** - Add 1 drop per 8 oz and stir
- **Sauces** - Add 1-2 drops and mix well

Supporting you now through your silver years, **Longevity Vitality**™ is a powerful blend that **provides overall wellness, care, and attention where you need it.**

- **Dressings** - Add 1-2 drops and shake to combine
- **Soups** - Stir in 1-2 drops
- **Cold Drinks** - Add 1 drop per 8 oz and stir
- **Sauces** - Add 1-2 drops and mix well
- **Dips** - Blend in 1-2 drops

Formulated for women, **SclarEssence™ Vitality**™ blends together a few of the top oils for **women's health** and support.

- **Dressings** - Add 1-2 drops and shake to combine
- **Soups** - Stir in 1-2 drops
- **Marinades** - Mix in 1-2 drops
- **Hot and Cold Drinks** - Add 1 drop per 8 oz and stir
- **Sauces** - Add 1-2 drops and mix well

Thieves Vitality™ is a great immune booster, but also adds delicious, spice and flavor to your favorite foods.

- **Soups** - Stir in 1-2 drops
- **Marinades** - Mix in 1-2 drops
- **Hot Drinks** - Add 1 drop per 8 oz and stir
- **Sauces** - Add 1-2 drops and mix well
- **Baked Goods** - Blend 1-2 drops into batter

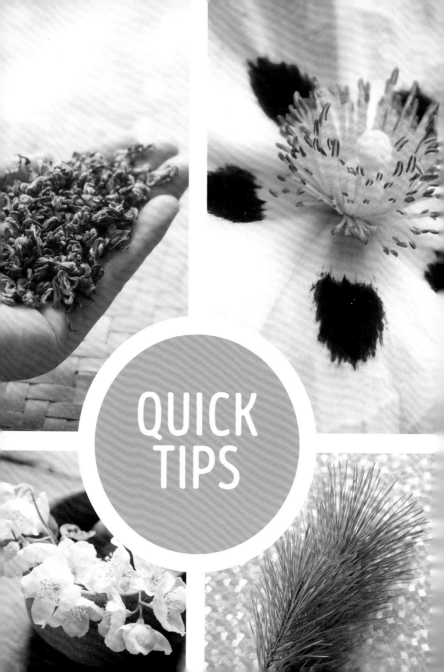

QUICK
TIPS

QUICK TIPS FOR OILS & BENEFITS

PROMOTE A HEALTHY EMOTIONAL STATE

Each essential oil boasts a complex, pleasant, and unique aroma that will activate the brain's center of emotion and memory (the limbic system) in a different way. Some essential oils may uplift your spirit; others help you release negative thoughts and habits. They can be very helpful as you strive for a healthier lifestyle and more balanced emotional state.

You can use the following oils and blends for diffusion, soothing baths, massage, inhalation, or topical application to help you rediscover peace, balance, and joy:

- Joy™
- Lavender
- Orange
- Peace & Calming®
- Peppermint
- Jasmine

IMPROVE YOUR PHYSICAL WELLNESS

Life gets busier and more chaotic each day, and your lifestyle doesn't always create an ideal opportunity to maintain physical wellness. Poor diet, lack of exercise, and being pummeled by environmental toxins can leave the body unbalanced. From cleansing and weight management to supporting all of the systems in your body, essential oils and essential oil-infused supplements, can provide the solutions you need.

Feel alive and refreshed every day with nutrients, powerful antioxidants, and pure essential oils found in these products:

- NingXia Red®
- Life 9™
- Slique® Tea
- OmegaGize3®
- Longevity™

CLEANSE YOUR HOME AND SURROUNDINGS

You don't have to use harsh chemicals to clean your home. You can polish countertops, remove sticky messes, repel bugs, and clean dirty areas with gentle and effective power of essential oils and Thieves® products.

There are convenient and non-chemical options for cleaning your home, without chemicals, leaving only pleasant scents and a healthy environment. You can replace the cleansers with these versatile products:

- Lemon
- Purification®
- Thyme
- Lemongrass
- Thieves® Household Cleaner

REFINE YOUR SKIN AND HAIR

Rediscover your natural glow and purge chemicals from your beauty routine. Essential oils can help soothe tension, support healthy cell growth, promote clear complexion, soften signs of aging, and nurture healthy hair. Here are some suggestions:

- ART® Renewal Serum
- Lavender
- Lavender Volume Shampoo/Conditioner
- Frankincense
- Copaiba Vanilla Shampoo/Conditioner
- Boswellia Wrinkle Cream™

PROMOTE SPIRITUAL AWARENESS

Incense and essential oils from plants have always had a starring role in religious and spiritual ceremonies, helping those involved to transcend the trivial and connect with something larger than themselves.

To enhance your spiritual experience, dilute and apply meditative, empowering essential oils directly to wrists, feet, and behind the ears, or diffuse in a quiet area. Popular oils and blends for spiritual focus include:

- Sacred Frankincense™
- White Angelica™
- Egyptian Gold™
- Inspiration™
- The Gift™

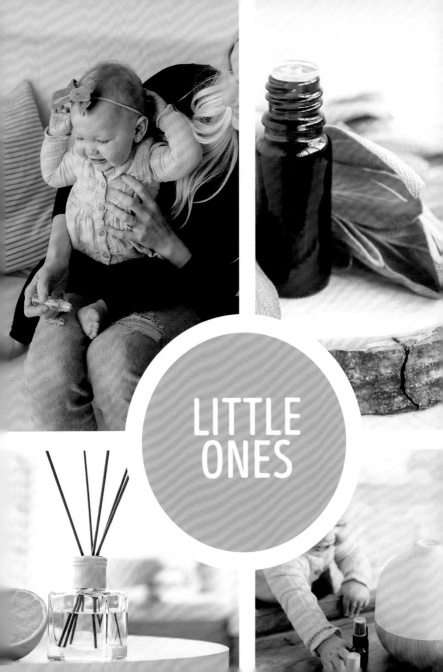

LITTLE
ONES

LITTLE ONES

Care for your little ones in the best way possible with natural, clean products from Young Living that you know you can trust.

BODY CARE

Rub-a-dub dub, KidScents® Bath Gel in your tub is a safe and gentle way to clean the kiddos with a neutral pH balance that is perfect for young skin. It contains no mineral oils, synthetic perfumes, artificial colorings, or toxic ingredients – just clean ingredients to help them get squeaky clean.

- Directions: Apply a small amount of KidScents® Bath Gel to washcloth or directly to the skin. Rub gently, then rinse.
- Ingredients: Water, Decyl Glucoside, Glycerin, Sorbitol, Dimethyl Sulfone (MSM), Roman Chamomile Flower Extract, Aloe Vera Leaf Juice, and more
- Essential Oils: Cedarwood, Geranium

Dry, itchy skin? That's no fun for anyone. KidScents® Lotion to the rescue with its safe, gentle, pH neutral, ingredients that are ideal for young skin. No mineral oils, synthetic perfumes, artificial colorings, or toxic ingredients means no worries and smooth, fresh skin for your little ones.

- Directions: Apply liberally to skin as needed.
- Ingredients: Water, Aloe Barbadensis Leaf Juice, Glycerin, Limnanthes Alba (Meadowfoam) Seed Oil, Pyrus Malus (Apple) Fruit Extract, and more
- Essential Oils: Tangerine, Lemon, Orange, Cedarwood, Coriander, Geranium, Bergamot, Ylang Ylang

Tangles and knots are not a problem for KidScents® Shampoo. Formulated for the most delicate hair, this mild formula provides the perfect pH balance for your children's hair and contains no mineral oils, synthetic perfumes, artificial colorings, or toxic ingredients that can dry or cause damage.

- Directions: Apply a small amount to hair. Lather, then rinse.
- Ingredients: Water, Decyl Glucoside, Dimethyl Sulfone (MSM), Roman Chamomile Flower Extract, Aloe Vera Leaf Juice, and more
- Essential Oils: Tangerine, Lemon

Make brushing a blast with KidScents® Toothpaste. This safe, natural alternative to commercial brands of toothpaste fights plaque and unwanted bad breath with a fluoride-free formula that tastes great and keeps young smiles bright!

- Directions: Put a small amount of toothpaste on a brush, help child brush teeth, and rinse thoroughly after each meal or as directed by a dentist or doctor. Do not swallow. Recommended for children two years or older.
- Ingredients: Water, Calcium Carbonate, Coconut Oil, Baking Soda (Sodium Bicarbonate), Vegetable Glycerin, Xylitol, Xanthan Gum, Stevia Leaf Extract
- Essential Oils: Grapefruit, Tangerine, Spearmint, Lemon, Ocotea, Clove, Cinnamon Bark, Eucalyptus Radiata, Rosemary

KidScents® Tender Tush™ is a gentle ointment designed to protect and nourish young skin and promote healing. This ointment soothes dry, chapped skin and offers protection for delicate skin. It is also great for expectant mothers who are concerned about stretch marks.

- Directions: Apply liberally to diaper area as often as needed to help soothe diaper rash, redness, or irritation.
- Ingredients: Coconut Oil, Cocoa Seed Butter, Olive Fruit Oil, Sweet Almond Oil, Beeswax, Wheat Germ Oil
- Essential Oils: Royal Hawaiian Sandalwood, Coriander, Roman Chamomile, Lavender, Frankincense, Bergamot (Furocoumarin-Free), Cistus, Ylang Ylang, Geranium

KIDSCENTS® NUTRITIONAL SUPPORT FOR CHILDREN

KidScents® MightyPro™ was created to boost your little one's digestive and immune health. With a delicious wolfberry punch flavor, this supplement delivers the power of both pre- and probiotics with over 8 billion active, live cultures of the friendly bacteria needed for optimal health.

- Directions: For children 2 years and above, empty entire content of 1 packet into mouth and allow it to dissolve. Take 1 packet daily with food to provide optimal conditions for healthy gut bacteria. Can be taken straight or combined with applesauce, yogurt, or other food or beverage. Do not add to warm or hot food or beverages.
- Ingredients: Fructooligosaccharides, Lactobacillus Paracasei Lpc-37, Lactobacillus Acidophilus LA-14, Goji Fruit Powder, Xylitol, and more

Super kids need serious super foods, but it's not always easy to pack them all in – especially with picky eaters! Make sure your kiddos are covered with KidScents® MightyVites™. Specifically designed for growing bodies, this whole food multinutrient contains super fruits, plants, and vegetables that deliver the full spectrum of vitamins, minerals, antioxidants, and phytonutrients that their bodies need to grow healthy and strong.

- Directions: Children ages 4-12, take 4 chewable tablets daily. Can be taken separately or in a single daily dose. Also available in chewable powder tablet with Wild Berry flavor.
- Ingredients: Vitamin A, Vitamin C (As Ascorbic Acid From Orange), Vitamin D (As Cholecalciferol), Vitamin E (As D-Alpha Tocopheryl Acid Succinate), and more

Missing vital enzymes? Not your kids! KidScents® MightyZyme™ is an all-natural, vegetarian, chewable tablet designed to give children added enzyme nutrition by combining nine different digestive enzymes with several other nutrients to support healthy digestion and relieve occasional symptoms— such as stomach pressure, bloating, gas, pain, and minor cramping—that may occur after eating.

- Directions: Take 1 tablet, 3 times daily, prior to or with meals.
- Ingredients: Calcium (From Calcium Carbonate), Lipase, Alfalfa (Medicago Sativa) Leaf Powder, Apple Juice Powder, and more
- Essential Oils: Peppermint

No more need for metaphorical "chill pills," KidScents® Unwind™ was created to help little ones settle down and enter a state of restfulness, focus, and peace.

- Directions: For children 4 years and older, empty contents of 1 packet into mouth and dissolve.
- Ingredients: Erythritol, Xylitol, Aquamin-Magnesium TG, Magnesium Citrate, L-Theanine, 5-HTP Griffonia Seed Extract, N-C Watermelon Flavor, and more
- Essential Oils: Lavender, Roman Chamomile

KIDSCENTS® OIL COLLECTION

Give your kid's brainpower a boost with KidScents® GeneYus™. This smart blend was fashioned specifically to help young minds focus and concentrate. Whether they are doing homework, reading a book, or learning a new skill, this grounding, calming blend will help block distractions and get them excited to learn and grow. Available in a Roll-On.

- Directions: Diffuse up to 1 hour, 3 times daily, or apply 2-4 drops directly to desired area - temples. Dilution not required except for the most sensitive skin.
- Ingredients: Caprylic/Capric Triglyceride, Almond Oil
- Essential Oils: Sacred Frankincense™, Blue Cypress, Cedarwood, Idaho Blue Spruce, Palo Santo, Melissa, Northern Lights Black Spruce, Bergamot, Myrrh, Vetiver, Geranium, Royal Hawaiian Sandalwood, Ylang Ylang, Hyssop, Rose

Bumps, bruises, scrapes, and scratches... KidScents® Owie™ has it covered! Cleansing and soothing properties come together in this MUST HAVE blend to greatly improve the appearance of your child's oopsies and ouchies. It also helps prevent infection to get your kid back out there in record time! Available in a Roll-On.

- Directions: Diffuse up to 1 hour, 3 times daily, or apply 2-4 drops directly to desired area. Dilution not required except for the most sensitive skin.
- Ingredients: Caprylic/Capric Triglyceride
- Essential Oils: Idaho Balsam Fir, Tea Tree, Helichrysum, Elemi, Cistus, Hinoki, Clove

Bedtime is a breeze with KidScents® SleepyIze™. Calming and comforting essential oils come together in this blend to help quiet and relax your littles mind and body prior to bedtime. Available in a Roll-On.

- Directions: Diffuse up to 1 hour, 3 times daily, or apply 2-4 drops directly to desired area - soles of feet or chest. Dilution not required except for the most sensitive skin.
- Ingredients: Caprylic/Capric Triglyceride
- Essential Oils: Lavender, Geranium, Roman Chamomile, Tangerine, Bergamot, Sacred Frankincense™, Valerian, Rue

Bless YOU! Caring for a congested child is no easy task. Luckily, KidScents® SniffleEase™ is here to help. This refreshing, rejuvenating blend was designed just for kids who are feeling stuffed up. This can help break through the blockage and soothe them through the sniffles. Available in a Roll-On.

- Directions: Diffuse up to 1 hour, 3 times daily, or apply 2-4 drops directly to desired area - chest or throat. Dilution not required except for the most sensitive skin.
- Ingredients: Caprylic/Capric Triglyceride
- Essential Oils: Eucalyptus Blue, Palo Santo, Lavender, Dorado Azul, Camphor, Eucalyptus Globulus, Myrtle, Marjoram, Pine, Eucalyptus Citriodora, Cypress, Eucalyptus Radiata, Northern Lights Black Spruce, Peppermint

KidScents® TummyGize™ takes on tummy troubles with a comforting blend that helps settle upset stomachs and support proper digestion.

- Directions: Diffuse up to 1 hour, 3 times daily, or apply 2-4 drops directly to desired area - stomach. Dilution not required except for the most sensitive skin.
- Ingredients: Caprylic/Capric Triglyceride
- Essential Oils: Spearmint, Peppermint, Tangerine, Fennel, Anise, Ginger, Cardamom

SEEDLINGS™ BABY PRODUCTS

Even silky-smooth baby skin needs to stay nourished. Seedlings™ Baby Lotion keeps your baby's skin soft and hydrated with all natural, plant-based ingredients that also help calm and relax your sweet little one.

- Directions: Apply a small amount to your hands. Rub hands together to warm the lotion and gently massage into baby's skin.
- Ingredients: Water, Caprylic/Capric Triglyceride, Glycerin, Glyceryl Stearate, Coco-Caprylate, Cetearyl Alcohol, Apple Fruit Extract, and more
- Essential Oils: Lavender, Coriander, Bergamot, Ylang Ylang, Geranium

Seedlings™ Baby Oil was specially crafted to care for your baby's delicate skin. No mineral oil or dangerous phthalates, means your baby's skin gets all its needed nourishment while providing the calming scent of appropriately diluted, pure essential oils.

- Directions: Apply a small amount to your hands. Rub hands together to warm the oil and gently massage into baby's skin.
- Ingredients: Caprylic/Capric Triglyceride, Apricot Kernel Oil, Safflower Seed Oil, Prickly Pear Seed Oil, Mixed Tocopherols
- Essential Oils: Lavender, Coriander, Bergamot (Furocoumarin-free), Ylang Ylang, Geranium

Gentle and mild for your baby's sensitive skin, Young Living's Seedlings™ Baby Wash & Shampoo is 100 percent plant based and free from harsh ingredients that can cause over drying. Not to mention the calming essential oil blend that adds a light and calming scent that soothes and enhances your baby's bathing experience.

- Directions: Wet hair and skin with warm water. Apply a small amount to a moistened washcloth or hand and gently lather over entire body and scalp.
- Ingredients: Water, Sodium Laurylglucosides Hydroxypropylsulfonate, Glycerin, Decyl Glucoside, Glyceryl Caprylate, Xanthan Gum, and more
- Essential Oils: Lavender, Coriander, Bergamot (Furocoumarin-free), Ylang Ylang, Geranium

Seedlings™ Baby Wipes soft, thick wipes are perfect for everything from a little spill to a not so little diaper change. The infused purifying botanical blend helps to clean and refresh without harsh chemicals. Dermatologist tested and hypoallergenic for worry-free care.

- Directions: Close lid firmly after each use to keep moist. Do not flush. Store at room temperature. **Caution:** To be applied only by a trusted adult. For external use only.
- Ingredients: Water, Glycerin, Phenethyl Alcohol, Apple Fruit Extract, Soapberry Fruit Extract, Marigold Flower Extract, Witch Hazel Leaf Extract, Caprylic/Capric Triglyceride, Aloe Vera Leaf Juice
- Essential Oils: Lavender, Coriander, Bergamot, Ylang Ylang, Geranium

Seedlings™ Diaper Cream is made with 100 percent naturally derived ingredients that provide extra-gentle protection. When used at the first sign of diaper rash, it can soothe irritation, protecting baby's tender skin and help heal the rash quickly.

- **Directions:** Change wet and soiled diapers promptly. Cleanse the diaper area and allow to dry. Apply cream liberally with each diaper change, especially at bedtime or anytime when exposure to wet diapers may be prolonged.
- **Ingredients:** non-nano zinc oxide, coconut oil, beeswax, castor oil, mango butter, sunflower oil, safflower oil, cocoa butter, and more
- **Essential Oils:** Lavender, Northern Lights Black Spruce, Helichrysum

Want fresh linens without the excessive washing? Crib sheets, blankets, even car seats can be freshened with the calming aroma of Seedlings™ Linen Spray. Not only does it leave your fabrics smelling fresh, it helps soothe and relax your little one.

- **Directions:** Shake well before each use. Spray on linens as needed. Do not spray directly on skin or face.
- **Ingredients:** water, glyceryl caprylate, glycerin, caprylyl/capryl glucoside, sodium levulinate, glyceryl undecylenate, and more
- **Essential Oils:** Lavender, Coriander, Bergamot, Ylang Ylang, Geranium

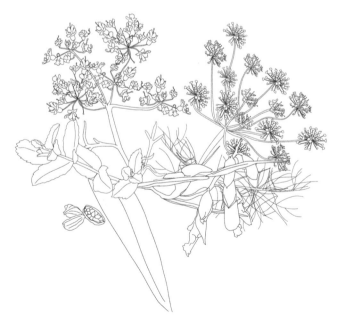

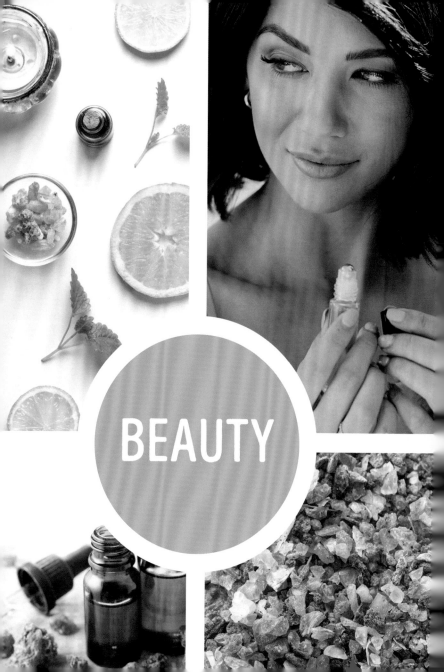

BEAUTY

BEAUTY

Beauty is all about confidence and what makes YOU feel your best – inside and out! Using all natural, clean products is just one way that you can ensure your true beauty shines through. Say no to harsh chemicals, and say yes to healthy, happy, glowing skin!

BLOOM™ BY YOUNG LIVING

Immerse your skin in BLOOM™ Brightening Essence for bright, dewy skin. Its pH balance-restoring formula aids in reducing the appearance of pores and fortifying your natural barriers for stronger, sleeker skin. Use it in combination with the BLOOM™ Brightening Cleanser and BLOOM™ Brightening Lotion to get a long-lasting luminous look and kiss dull skin goodbye.

- Directions: Gently shake before use. Pour a quarter-sized amount into palms. Rub hands together and lightly press palms into skin from the center of face outward, including neck and décolletage. Repeat morning and night.
- Ingredients: Aqua/Water/Eau, Glycerin, Pyrus Malus (Apple) Fruit Extract, Sea Water/Eau De Mer, Levulinic Acid, Xanthan Gum, Benzoic Acid, Glycyrrhiza Glabra (Licorice) Root Extract, and more
- Essential Oils: Vetiver, Blue Cypress, Davana, Royal Hawaiian Sandalwood™, Clove, Carrot, Jasmine, Spearmint, Geranium, Sacred Frankincense™

Brighten your skin, and your morning, with Young Living's BLOOM™ Brightening Cleanser. It goes beyond cleansing to purifying so your best skin shines through.

- Directions: Wet skin with lukewarm water and gently massage a small amount of cleanser onto skin. Rinse thoroughly and pat dry, repeating both morning and night.
- Ingredients: Aqua (Water), Disodium Cocoyl Glutamate, Decyl Glucoside, Glycerin, Sodium Laurylglucosides Hydroxypropylsulfonate, and more
- Essential Oils: Vetiver, Blue Cypress, Davana, Royal Hawaiian Sandalwood™, Clove, Carrot, Spearmint, Geranium, Sacred Frankincense™

BLOOM™ Brightening Lotion by Young Living highlights your natural beauty by helping to brighten and hydrate your skin. Its lightweight formula makes it ideal for saturating into skin to reach and moisturize your deepest layers.

- **Directions:** Gently press and pat two pumps of lotion evenly over face, neck, and decolletage. Repeat morning and night.
- **Ingredients:** Aqua/Water/Eau, Glycerin, Caprylic/capric triglyceride, Glyceryl stearates, Sodium stearoyl lactylate, Plumeria acutifolia flower extract, and more
- **Essential Oils:** Vetiver, Blue Cypress, Davana, Royal Hawaiian Sandalwood™, Clove, Jasmine, Carrot, Spearmint, Geranium, Sacred Frankincense™
-

ART®

The ART® Refreshing Toner combines a blend of cleansing and tightening essential oils to clear your skin without drying. Its unique formula helps balance your skin's pH and remove excess contaminations- leaving your face clean, toned, and energized. Use the ART Refreshing Toner in combination with the ART Gentle Cleanser to remove impurities and leave your skin rejuvenated.

- **Directions:** After cleansing skin, sweep toner across face and neck with a cotton ball. Use morning and evening as needed.
- **Ingredients:** Water, Alcohol, Heptyl glucoside, Hamamelis virginiana (Witch hazel) water, Glycerin, Betaine, Orchis mascula flower extract, Aloe barbadensis leaf juice, Camellia sinensis (Green tea) leaf extract
- **Essential Oils:** Peppermint, Royal Hawaiian Sandalwood™, Sacred Frankincense™, Lavender, Lemon, Melissa

An intricate blend of orchid extract and nourishing essential oils, the **ART® Renewal Serum** deeply permeates, hydrates, and replenishes your skin to help maintain a youthful appearance. Use in the morning to smooth your skin and create an even surface or apply before bed to lock in moisture and saturate overnight. Use morning or night. Safe and recommended for all skin types.

- **Directions:** Wash face. Apply ART® Renewal Serum to delicate areas of face, 2 times daily, and allow to absorb. For best results, follow up with your choice of Young Living's moisturizing creams.
- **Ingredients:** (Water) Aqua, Glycerin, Selaginella Lepidophylla Extract, Lactobacillus Ferment, Speranskia Tuberculate (Snow Lotus) Whole Plant Extract, Proprietary Young Living Sensation Essential Oil Blend, and more
- **Essential Oils:** Coriander, Ylang Ylang, Bergamot, Jasmine, Geranium

Long days and stress leaving you with a dreary complexion? ART® Sheerlumé™ is here to help! An advanced formula powered by a sophisticated and exclusive blend of alpine botanicals and pure essential oils, Sheerlumé™ will visibly brighten and balance skin tones to help you have more luminous, beautiful skin- naturally.

- Directions: Apply a thin layer of Sheerlumé™ on clean skin—face, neck, or hands. For best results, use morning and night either alone or under your favorite Young Living® moisturizing cream.
- Ingredients: Water (Aqua), Glycerin, Coconut Alkanes, Caprylic/Capric Triglycerides, Theobroma Grandiflorum Seed Butter, and more
- Essential Oils: Vetiver, Blue Cypress, Davana, Royal Hawaiian Sandalwood™, Clove, Jasmine, Carrot, Spearmint, Geranium, Sacred Frankincense™

YOUNG LIVING SPECIALTY CARE

A fresh, clear complexion is yours with the help of Young Living's® Maximum-Strength Acne Treatment. Naturally derived, maximum-strength salicylic acid from Wintergreen helps clear acne blemishes, pimples, and blackheads; but its plant-based powers don't stop there! Some acne treatments leave skin feeling tight and dry, but with the addition of aloe and chamomile extracts, Young Living's® Maximum-Strength Acne Treatment fights blemishes while keeping skin soft, smooth, and moisturized.

- Directions: Cover the entire affected area with a thin layer, 1-3 times daily. If bothersome dryness or peeling occurs, reduce application to 1 time a day or every other day.
- Ingredients: Salicylic Acid 2 percent, Water, Aloe Vera Leaf, Lactovacillus Reuteri, Coconut Alkanes, Sunflower Oil, Chamomile, Saliz Alba Bark, and more
- Essential Oils: Manuka, Frankincense, Rosemary, Geranium, Tea Tree (Melaleuca Alternifolia), Lavender

Wolfberry Eye Cream is a natural, water-based moisturizer formulated for the delicate skin in the eye area. Containing the anti-aging and skin-conditioning properties of wolfberry seed oil, this cream soothes tired eyes and minimizes the appearance of fine lines.

- Directions: After cleansing and toning, massage gently onto soft skin under the eyes. Use in the evening.
- Ingredients: Deionized Water, Sorbitol, Glycerin, Cetearyl Alcohol, Glyceryl Stearate, Sodium Stearoyl Lactylate, Oat Kernal Extract, Camellia Sinensis (Green Tea) Leaf Extract, and more.
- Essential Oils: Lavender, Coriandrum, Roman Chamomile, Frankincense, Geranium, Bergamot, Ylang Ylang

SAVVY® MINERALS

Get primed to glow with Savvy Minerals by Young Living® Mattifying Primer. This silky-smooth formula helps blur and smooth fine lines while providing an even surface for foundation to adhere to – extending the wear of your makeup.

- Directions: Apply a thin, even layer to clean, moisturized skin. Allow a few minutes for the primer to set before applying makeup.
- Ingredients: Water, Caprylic/Capric Triglyceride, Steraryl Alcohol, Cetearyl Alcohol, Silica, Kaolin, Prunus Amygdalus Dulcis (Sweet Almond) Oil, and more
- Essential Oils: Manuka, Tea Tree (Melaleuca Alternifolia), Geranium, Lavender, Frankincense, Rosemary

Girl, Savvy Minerals by Young Living® Liquid Foundation has you covered. Formulated as a medium- to full-coverage foundation, it provides a natural, clean foundation you can build on, and a foundation you can trust.
Available in shades: Porcelain, Buff, Fresh Beige, Natural Beige, Sand Beige, Honey, Tan, Caramel, Truffle, Pecan, Cocoa, Ivory, Hazelnut

- Directions: Shake bottle before use. For medium coverage, apply a small amount from the center of the face outward and blend with fingertips. For fuller coverage, use the Savvy Minerals Full-Coverage Foundation Brush to build and layer as needed, and use Savvy Minerals Powder Foundation to create and set a matte, long-lasting wear.
- Ingredients: Water, C15-19 alkane, Coconut alkanes, Glycerin, Polyglyceryl-6 polyricinoleate, Caprylic/capric triglyceride, Polyglyceryl-3 diisostearate, Cellulose (natural polymer), Persea gratissima (Avocado) oil, and more
- Essential Oils: Sacred Sandalwood

Breathable, buildable, beautiful coverage is at your brush tip with Savvy Minerals® Foundation Powder. This clean, mineral-based formula is easy to apply, and gives you options from sheer to full coverage that lasts all day.
Available in shades: Cool NO 1-3, Warm NO 1-3, Dark NO 1

- Directions: Sprinkle a small amount of Foundation into the jar lid and swirl the brush in the lid to collect the powder. Lightly tap the brush handle to dust off any excess. Using circular motions, blend the Foundation onto your skin, repeating to build coverage. For more controlled coverage, spritz your brush, 2–3 times with Savvy Minerals Misting Spray before swirling in the powder.
- Ingredients: Mica, Boron Nitride, Lauroyl Lysine, Populus Tremuloides (Aspen) Bark Extract, Kaolin Clay, Silica

Blemishes, dark circles, pigment, oh my! Made with clean, naturally derived ingredients, Savvy Minerals Liquid Concealer helps cover spots, lighten the look of undereye circles, and hide the <u>very few</u> imperfections you may see, while also smoothing and hydrating your skin.

Available in shades: Light 1-2, Medium 1-2, Dark 1-2

- **Directions:** Shake well before use. Apply concealer directly onto blemishes or imperfections and blend with the fingertips, a sponge or brush. To cover and conceal dark circles, apply 3 dots under the eye area, focusing on where the color is most intense. Blend outward.
- **Ingredients:** Water, C15-19 Alkane, Polyglyceryl-10 Pentaisostearate, Polyglyceryl-6 polyricinoleate, Polyglyceryl-3 diisostearate, Sodium Chloride, Glycerin, Persea Gratissima (Avocado) Oil, and more
- **Essential Oils:** Manuka, Tea Tree (Melaleuca Alternifolia)

Spritz, spritz.... and done! You've now got a flawless finish to your makeup masterpiece. Made with pure essential oils, trace minerals, and entirely plant-based ingredients, Savvy Minerals by Young Living® Misting Spray nourishes and freshens your skin for better coverage and all-day wear.

- **Directions:** Spray 2-3 pumps onto skin after applying makeup for longer lasting results. For powder foundation, Spray 2–3 pumps onto a makeup brush and gently wipe off any excess moisture. Pick up mineral makeup using the brush. Apply mineral makeup to your face in desired area and reapply as needed.
- **Ingredients:** Water, Glycerin, Aloe Barbadensis (Aloe Vera) Leaf Juice, Potassium Sorbate, Sodium Levulinate, Sodium Anisate, Trace Mineral Complex, Vanilla Planifolia (Vanilla) Fruit Extract
- **Essential Oils:** Geranium, Bergamot, Balsam Copaiba, Cedarwood, Black Spruce, Orange, Lavender, Lime, Sage, Ocotea, Rose

Want to look sun-kissed without the sunburn? Enhance your natural beauty and get that natural glow any time of year with the Savvy Minerals by Young Living® Mineral Bronzer Powder. Create all-over warmth while achieving a sculpted or contoured look with this long-lasting, buildable powder.

Available in shades: Crowned All Over, Summer Loved

- **Directions:** After applying foundation, sprinkle a small amount of bronzer onto its jar lid. Dip the brush into the lid to pick up the powder, then lightly tap the brush handle against the side of the lid to remove the excess. Apply bronzer to areas of the face where the sun hits naturally, including cheekbones, bridge of nose, forehead, and chin. Build color gradually to avoid overapplication.
- **Ingredients:** Mica, Populus Tremuloides (Aspen) Bark Extract

The **Savvy Minerals by Young Living® Mineral Blush** adds a natural-looking flush to your cheeks with clean, talc-free, mineral-based ingredients to provide the look you want from beautifully natural to daringly dramatic.

Available in shades: Smashing, Passionate, Awestruck, Captivate, Charisma, I Do Believe You're Blushin'

- **Directions:** After applying foundation, sprinkle a small amount of blush onto its jar lid. Dip the brush into the lid to pick up the powder, then lightly tap the brush handle against the side of the lid to remove the excess. Apply blush to the apples of the cheeks and blend outward, along the cheekbone toward the temples. Build color gradually to avoid over-application.
- **Ingredients:** Mica, Populus Tremuloides (Aspen) Bark Extract, Kaolin Clay

Want to add a little wow? How about an even bigger WOW? **Savvy Minerals by Young Living® Mineral Eyeliner** allows you to control and achieve a subtle or high-impact eye. Made with mineral-based ingredients, talc and paraben free, it is an ideal eyeliner for sensitive skin and can be used wet or dry to achieve desired intensity.

- **Directions:** Tap desired amount of powder into the cap, dip the brush in the powder, then lightly tap the brush handle against the side of the lid to remove the excess. Starting at the inside corner of the eye, apply the powder over the top of the lash line, moving outward. For a smokey look, apply the eyeliner dry and then smudge it with a sponge-tip applicator or cotton swab. For a higher-impact, liquid look, apply the eyeliner powder wet. Tap desired amount of powder into the cap or on a mixing surface. Mix a few drops of water into the powder with the eyeliner brush, then apply along the lash line.
- **Ingredients:** Mica, Populus Tremuloides (Aspen) Bark Extract, Kaolin Clay

Savvy Minerals by Young Living® Eyeshadow is all about the *drama* – in a good way! These rich shades are made with a finely ground mineral base and high-quality ingredients that make application smooth and easy, so the only drama you have is deciding how much to add.

Available in shades: Best Kept Secret (Matte), Wanderlust, Residual, Freedom, Inspired, Envy, Overboard

- **Directions:** Dip the brush into the eyeshadow powder, then lightly tap the brush handle against the side of the lid to remove the excess. Apply lightly to eyelids, building and blending color as desired.
- **Ingredients:** Mica, Populus Tremuloides (Aspen) Bark Extract

Savvy Minerals by Young Living® MultiTasker™ is your type I best friend that can do it all! Richly pigmented, this deep brown shade works perfectly as an eyeliner, eyeshadow, or brow filler. Its fine texture blends beautifully for smooth, even, and buildable application that will last you all day.

Available in shades: Regular, Dark

- Directions: Dip the brush into the MultiTasker powder, then lightly tap the brush handle against the side of the lid to remove the excess. Apply lightly where needed, building and blending color as desired.
- Ingredients: Mica, Populus Tremuloides (Aspen) Bark Extract

Looking for a mascara that works with sensitive eyes? We've got you covered. Savvy Minerals by Young Living® Mascara lets you flutter your lashes with confidence! This mascara complements a subtle daytime look or a fun evening style with natural definition.

Available in formulas: Sensitive, Volumizing, Lengthening

- Directions: Apply mascara from the roots of the lashes to the tips on upper and lower lashes. Wiggle wand while using an upward stroke to deposit extra product. For best results, allow mascara to dry between additional applications to build extra volume and length.
- Ingredients: Water, Glycerin, Hydroxystearic/Linolenic/Oleic Polyglycerides, Beeswax, Citric acid, Cocos Nucifera(Coconut) Fruit Extract, Sodium Hydroxide, and more
- Essential Oils: Lavender, Rosemary (Volumizing), Cedarwood (Volumizing)

Savvy Minerals by Young Living® Lip Gloss soothes and softens lips while adding shine and color without synthetic colorants. Its naturally derived, buildable tint gives you perfect control over your shade for sheer to medium color.

Available in shades: Abundant, Embrace, Maven, Rockin', Anchors Aweigh, Headliner

- Directions: Apply over the lips alone or with your favorite Savvy Minerals by Young Living Lipstick.
- Ingredients: Ricinus Communis (Castor) Seed Oil, Oleic/Linoleic/Linolenic Polyglycerides, Beeswax, Olea Europaea (Olive) Fruit Oil, Helianthus Annuus (Sunflower) Seed Oil, Silica, Jojoba Esters, Tocopheryl Acetate, Tocopherol
- Essential Oils: Peppermint

Made without synthetic colorants, Savvy Minerals® Lipstick adds a pop of color with a weightless formula, buildable color, and smooth application for a no-fuss lipstick that's perfect for everyday use.

Available in shades: Wish, Adore, Uptown Girl

- Directions: Moisturize lips with Young Living lip balm, then apply lipstick to lips until preferred level of coverage is reached.
- Ingredients: Ricinus Communis (Castor) Seed Oil, Prunus Amygdalus Dulcis (Sweet Almond) Oil, Euphorbia Cerifera (Candelilla) Wax, Beeswax, Tocopheryl

The Savvy Minerals Brush Set has you covered with a cute carrying case and five essential makeup application brushes designed to hold the optimal amount of product. The set includes a Foundation Brush to buff out your base, a Blush Brush perfect for creating rosy cheeks, an Eyeshadow Brush to elevate your eyes, a Veil Brush to softly dust your face with shimmer, and a Blending Brush to bring it all together.

Set includes: Blending Brush, Blush Brush, Eyeshadow Brush, Foundation Brush, Veil Brush, Carrying Case

Kabuki Brush:

Made with luxurious, high-quality, densely packed bristles, **Savvy Mineral's Kabuki Makeup Brush** offers controlled coverage and beautiful blending with a heavenly feel your skin will love.

Contour Brush:

Fear the contour no more. **The Savvy Minerals Contour Brush** makes it simple and easy to get the cut and carved look you want.

Concealer Brush:

Pinpoint and cover up imperfections on your skin with the **Savvy Minerals Concealer Brush.** Its compact size and packed bristles make it easy to apply the right amount of coverage for your needs.

Bronzer Brush:

Angled to give you more precise shading, the **Savvy Minerals Bronzer Brush** easily sweeps across your face turning you into a bronzed babe in no time.

Eyebrow Brush:

Dual sided, the **Savvy Minerals Eyebrow Brush** combs eyebrows then flips to apply the perfect amount of product to make your eyebrows really stand out.

Eyeliner Brush:

Savvy Mineral's Eyeliner Brush is there for you through thick and thin. Dual sided, its pinpoint edge allows for perfect precision while its thicker, angled side gives you full controlled coverage.

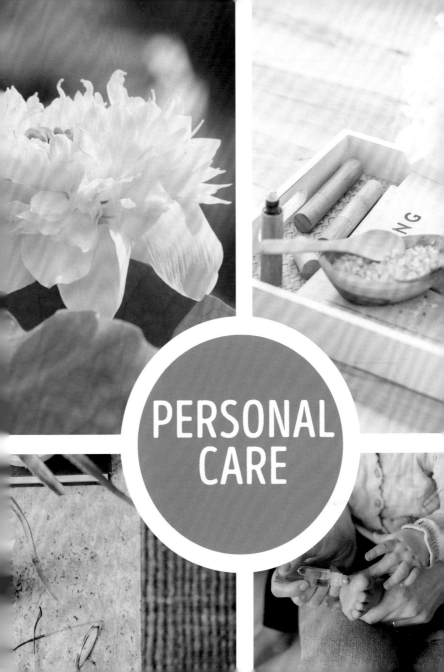

PERSONAL
CARE

PERSONAL CARE

Living a healthy lifestyle is much more than just what you put into your body! It's also what you put ON your body and how you choose to take care of yourself. Even with the busiest schedules, personal care can double as important self-care time that your body needs to be its best.

HAIR CARE

Luscious, healthy hair is just a bottle away with the **Copaiba Vanilla Moisturizing Shampoo**. Ultra-hydrating ingredients add shine to hair for a glowing sheen that looks and feels great.

- **Directions:** Use daily to hydrate dry or damaged hair.
- **Ingredients:** Water, Decyl Glucoside, Coco Betaine, Lauryl Glucoside, Coco-Glucoside, Glyceryl Oleate, Sorbitan Sesquicaprylate, Glycerin, and more
- **Essential Oils:** Lavender, Copaiba, Geranium

Copaiba Vanilla Moisturizing Conditioner enriches and hydrates dry, damaged hair providing you with softer, healthier hair.

- **Directions:** Use daily to hydrate dry or damaged hair.
- **Ingredients:** Water, Cetearyl Alcohol, Behenamidopropyl Dimethylamine, Glyceryl Stearate, Glycerin, Levulinic Acid, p-Anisic Acid, and more
- **Essential Oils:** Lavender, Copaiba, Geranium

Using **Lavender Mint Daily Shampoo** is an experience in the shower. Not only are you nourishing your hair, you are also creating a moment of important self-care! The crisp, naturally derived mint invigorates and nourishes the scalp while the lavender carries your stress down the drain- leaving you feeling relaxed and your hair looking fab.

- **Directions:** Use daily to cleanse and nourish hair.
- **Ingredients:** Water, Decyl Glucoside, Coco-Betaine, Lauryl Glucoside, Sorbitan Sesquicaprylate, Behenamidopropyl Dimethylamine, Lactic Acid, Glycerin, Inulin, Coco-Glucoside, Glyceryl Oleate, Xanthan Gum, and more
- **Essential Oils:** Peppermint, Lavender, Spearmint

Lavender Mint Daily Conditioner is your second step to having healthy, happy hair and a calmed mind. The invigorating scent promotes feelings of calm and clarity while nourishing ingredients create beautiful, strong, hydrated hair.

- **Directions:** Use daily to lightly condition and nourish hair.

- **Ingredients:** Water, Cetearyl Alcohol, Glycerin, Behenamidopropyl Dimethylamine, Glyceryl Stearate, Lactic Acid, and more
- **Essential Oils:** Peppermint, Lavender, Spearmint

Hair feeling a little flat? Use Young Living's **Lavender Volume Shampoo** to gently cleanse and nourish fine hair. The added botanical extracts, vitamins, and essential oils work to remove buildup that weighs hair down while maximizing body.

- **Directions:** Use daily to cleanse and strengthen hair.
- **Ingredients:** Cocos Nucifera (Coconut) Oil, Olea Europaea (Olive) Fruit Oil, Decyl Glucoside, Dimethyl Sulfone (MSM), Water, PEG-8 Dimethicone, Glycine Soja (Soybean) Protein, and more
- **Essential Oils:** Lavender, Clary Sage, Lemon

Fight flat hair with Young Living's **Lavender Volume Conditioner.** Formulated with all-natural ingredients, it works hard to gently hydrate and smooth fine hair without weighing it down. When combined with Lavender Shampoo, Lavender Conditioner provides shine and extra body to fine hair that otherwise falls flat.

- **Directions:** Use daily to cleanse and strengthen hair.
- **Ingredients:** Vegetable Fatty Acid Base, Dimethyl Sulfone (MSM), Quinoa (Chenopodium Quinoa) Extract, Milk Protein, and more
- **Essential Oils:** Lavender, Clary Sage, Lemon, Jasmine

DENTAL CARE

Show off your dazzling smile with **Thieves® AromaBright™ Toothpaste.** This all-natural recipe is tough on buildup, but gentle on teeth and enamel so your pearly whites can take center stage.

- **Directions:** Apply toothpaste to brush, brush teeth, and rinse thoroughly after each meal or as directed by a dentist or doctor. Do not swallow. For children under 2 years of age, consult a dentist or doctor before use.
- **Ingredients:** Water, Calcium Carbonate, Cocos Nucifera (Coconut) Oil, Sodium Bicarbonate, Glycerin, Xylitol, Xanthan Gum, and more
- **Essential Oils:** Peppermint, Spearmint, Clove, Ocotea, Cinnamon Bark, Lemon, Eucalyptus Radiata, Rosemary

Double fibers and double essential oils mean double the protection for your teeth. **Thieves® Dental Floss** was created with strong, fray resistant string, and infused with the signature Thieves® blend to help you get those hard-to-reach places and keep your gums and teeth strong.

- **Directions:** Floss teeth at least once daily, additionally as needed.
- **Ingredients:** Microcrystalline Wax
- **Essential Oils:** Clove, Cinnamon Bark, Lemon, Eucalyptus Radiata, Rosemary, Peppermint

Need fresh breath ASAP?! Alcohol and fluoride free, **Thieves® Fresh Essence Plus™** Mouthwash cleans hard-to-reach areas of the teeth and gums for a whole-mouth clean that leaves you feeling fresh.

- **Directions:** Rinse mouth with 1 tablespoon or capful of Thieves Fresh Essence Plus Mouthwash for 30-60 seconds or as needed.
- **Ingredients:** Water, Colloidal Silver, Lecithin, Quillaja Saponaria Wood Extract, Potassium Sorbate, Stevia Rebaudiana (Stevia) Leaf Extract, Tocopheryl, Citric Acid
- **Essential Oils:** Peppermint, Clove, Spearmint, Lemon, Cinnamon Bark, Vetiver, Eucalyptus Radiata, Rosemary

BODY CARE

A must have in your home, **Cool Azul® Sports Gel** is not just for ultra-competitors. The cooling effect of the essential oils combined with the quick absorption gel offers fast-acting relief from minor muscle and joint aches caused from just being human.

- **Directions:** Shake well before use. Rub and massage generously into skin. Wash hands after use.
- **Ingredients:** Methyl Salicylate, Aloe Barbadensis (Aloe Vera) Leaf Extract, Carthamus Tinctorius (Safflower) Seed oil, Gylcerul Monostearate, Cetyl Alcohol, and more
- **Essential Oils:** Wintergreen, Peppermint, Sage, Oregano, Niaouli, Lavender, Blue Cypress, Elemi, Vetiver, Dorado Azul, Roman Chamomile

Need a minute for yourself? Unwind with a luxurious **Dream Catcher™ Bath Bomb** in warm comforting water. Infused with a combination of fresh, floral, and slightly citrus scents, this deluxe bath bomb helps you relax and refresh.

- **Directions:** Drop bath bomb into tub filled with warm water, then lie back, relax, and visualize your dreams coming true.
- **Ingredients:** Sodium bicarbonate, Citric acid, Water/aqua, Cocos nucifera (Coconut) oil, Prunus amygdalus dulcis (Sweet Almond) oil, Maltodextrin, Ultramarine, and more
- **Essential Oils:** Sandalwood, Tangerina, Ylang Ylang, Bergamot, Anise, Juniper, Geranium, Blue Cypress, Davana, Kaffir Lime, Roman Chamomile, Grapefruit, Spearmint, Lemon, Ocotea

Spending time in the great outdoors is so much fun, but insect bites are not! Keep the bugs away with Young Living's natural, essential oil-infused **Insect Repellent.** Free of harsh chemicals, this powerful recipe works effectively to prevent mosquito, flea, and tick bites.

- **Directions:** Dispense into hand and apply evenly over exposed skin. Reapply as needed. Avoid contact with clothing, as product can stain fabric.
- **Ingredients:** Sesame Oil, Vitamin E
- **Essential Oils:** Citronella, Lemongrass, Rosemary, Geranium, Spearmint, Thyme, Clove

Need serious sun protection? Young Living's **SPF 50 Mineral Sunscreen Lotion** offers powerful defense against UVA and UVB rays without the harsh ingredients found in other sunscreens.

- **Directions:** Apply liberally 15 minutes before sun exposure. Reapply after 80 minutes of swimming or sweating, immediately after towel drying, or after 2 hours of wear.
- **Ingredients:** Zinc Oxide, Caprylic/Capric Triglycerid, Beeswax, Rininus Communis (Castor) Seed Oil, Coco-Caprylate/Caprate, Cocos Nucifera (Coconut) Oil, Helianthus Annuus (Sunflower) Seed Oil, and more
- **Essential Oils:** Helichrysum, Lavender, Myrrh, Cistus, Ylang Ylang, Carrot Seed, Sacred Frankincense™

Aluminum-free AromaGuard® Mountain Mint™ Deodorant harnesses all-natural ingredients like coconut oil, beeswax, vitamin E, and pure essential oils that keep you smelling fresh all day long without harmful chemicals found in commercial products.

- **Directions:** Apply daily to underarms.
- **Ingredients:** Cocos Nucifera (Coconut) Oil Extract, White Beeswax, Pure Ester 34, Zinc Oxide, Pure Ester 40, Tocopherol (Vitamin E)
- **Essential Oils:** Clove, Lemon, Peppermint, Rosemary, Eucalyptus Radiata, White Fir

Citrus Fresh™ Energizing Shower Steamers are the best way to start your day! Simply place one or two steamers on the floor of your shower, or on the shelf opposite your shower head, and instantly be surrounded by the energizing and empowering aroma of citrus and spearmint.

- **Directions:** Place 1 shower steamer onto the shower floor or shelf where it gets wet but does not obstruct the main water stream. Breathe in the fragrant steam for an amazing, spa-like experience.
- **Ingredients:** Sodium bicarbonate, Sodium sesquicarbonate, Citric acid, Water, Maltodextrin, Carthamus tinctorius (Safflower) seed oil
- **Essential Oils:** Orange, Tangerine, Grapefruit, Lemon, Mandarin, Spearmint

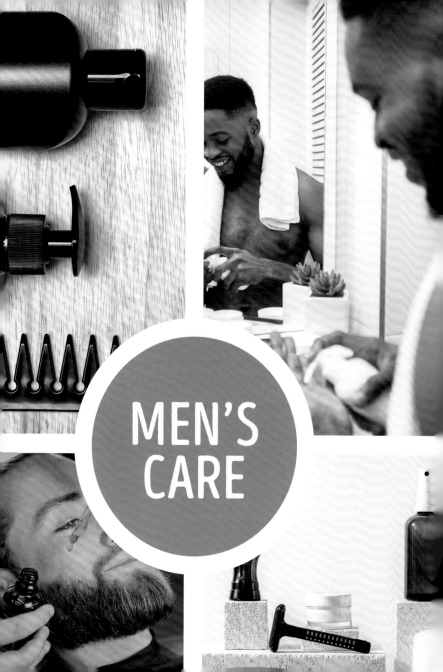

MEN'S
CARE

MEN'S CARE

Shutran 3-in-1 Men's Wash saves shower space and cleans from head to toe–literally! One wash to rule them all–Shutran takes care of hair, body, and face with fresh, cleansing essential oils and other nature made ingredients.

- **Directions:** Lather over hair, body, and face. Rinse.
- **Ingredients:** Water, Decyl Glucoside, Glycerin, Sodium Lauryl Glucosides Hydroxypropylsulfonate, PCA Glyceryl Oleate, Xanthan Gum, and more
- **Essential Oils:** Idaho Blue Spruce, Ylang Ylang, Ocotea, Hinoki, Davana, Cedarwood, Lavender, Coriander, Lemon, Northern Lights Black Spruce

The perfect post-shave companion, **Shutran Aftershave Lotion** helps seal hydration into the skin after shaving and reduces inflammation–leaving skin comfortable, soft, and smooth.

- **Directions:** Apply a small amount to face after shaving with Young Living's Shutran Shave Cream. Can also be applied between shaves to keep skin moisturized.
- **Ingredients:** Water, Glycerin, Caprylic/capric triglyceride, Simmondsia chinensis (Jojoba) seed oil, Cocos nucifera (Coconut) oil, Polyglyceryl-10 pentastearate, and more
- **Essential Oils:** Idaho Blue Spruce, Ylang Ylang, Ocotea, Hinoki, Davana, Cedarwood, Lemon, Coriander, Lavender, Northern Lights Black Spruce

Skin-nourishing ingredients, essential oils, and activated carbon all come together to play in the **Shutran Soap Bar**. Perfect for an all over scrubbing and detoxing wash that will leave you feeling fresh and clean.

- **Directions:** Wet bar and work into a lather. Apply lather to desired areas of the body to cleanse skin. Rinse thoroughly with water.
- **Ingredients:** Sodium palmate, Sodium palm kernelate, Water, Glycerin, Olea europaea (Olive) fruit oil, Butyrospermum parkii (Shea) butter, Sodium gluconate, Lycium barbarum (Wolfberry) seed oil, and more
- **Essential Oils:** Idaho Blue Spruce, Ylang Ylang, Ocotea, Hinoki, Davana, Cedarwood, Lavender, Coriander, Lemon, Northern Lights Black Spruce

Love the beard but hate how rough it is? **Shutran® Beard Oil** is for you! Designed with pure ingredients that easily absorb into hair, this beard oil will leave your skin hydrated and your beard softer than ever before.

- **Directions:** Use the dropper to dispense a dime-sized amount of oil into the palm of your hand. Gently work the oil into your facial hair. Groom and style your facial hair as normal. Rinse excess oil from your hands with warm, soapy water.
- **Ingredients:** Caprylic/capric triglyceride, Helianthus annuus (Sunflower) seed oil, Prunus armeniaca (Apricot) kernel oil, Lycium barbarum (Wolfberry) seed oil, Tocopherol
- **Essential Oils:** Idaho Blue Spruce, Ylang Ylang, Ocotea, Hinoki, Davana, Cedarwood, Lavender, Coriander, Lemon, Northern Lights Black Spruce

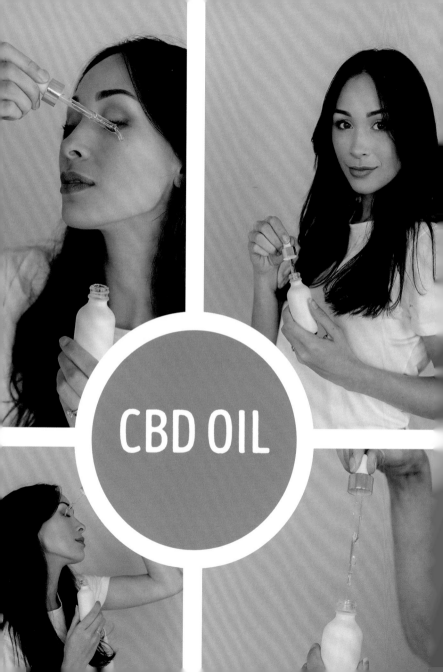

CBD OIL

CBD

From battling aches and pains to improving concentration and relaxation, CBD has the power to take on every day human issues in a natural way. Nature's Ultra CBD takes those benefits to the next level by pairing it with the power of your essential oils for even more amazing results. Time to see what it can do for you!

Feeling tired or stressed after a long day, but can't seem to relax? Take a load off with the **Calm CBD Roll-On**. Formulated to help you find your peace, this valuable combination of CBD and relaxing essential oils will help quiet your mind and chill.

- **Directions:** Apply generously to chest and neck as desired.
- Proprietary carrier oil blend (Apricot kernel oil, Argan oil, Avocado oil, Camellia seed oil, Evening primrose oil, Hemp seed oil, Neem oil, Rosehip seed oil, Sweet almond oil), Cannabidiol (CBD - 0.0 percent THC)
- **Essential Oils:** Lavender, Vetiver, Eucalyptus Globulus, Frankincense, Orange, Ylang Ylang

Nature's Ultra Cinnamon CBD Oil combines potent CBD with the anti-inflammatory power of Cinnamon Bark essential oil to help cleanse and combat irritation in your body.

- **Directions:** Apply one full dropper to desired area. Shake well before use. Keep in a cool, dry place.
- **Ingredients:** MCT coconut oil, Cannabidiol (CBD - 0.0 percent THC), Organic stevia leaf extract
- **Essential Oils:** Cinnamon Bark

Nature's Ultra Citrus CBD Oil is your best friend when the blues hit. Energizing and uplifting, this powerful blend of CBD with Orange and Grapefruit essential oils helps you wake up, stay up, and show up so you can conquer the day!

- **Directions:** Apply one full dropper to desired area. Shake well before use. Keep in a cool, dry place.
- **Ingredients:** MCT coconut oil, Cannabidiol (CBD - 0.0 percent THC), Organic stevia leaf extract
- **Essential Oils:** Grapefruit, Orange

Focus up with **Nature's Ultra Cool Mint CBD Oil**. In this powerful blend, CBD's natural ability to calm combines with the uplifting and focusing benefits of Spearmint and Peppermint to refresh and invigorate you on even the busiest days.

- **Directions:** Apply one full dropper to desired area. Shake well before use. Keep in a cool, dry place.
- **Ingredients:** MCT coconut oil, Cannabidiol (CBD - 0.0 percent THC), Organic stevia leaf extract
- **Essential Oils:** Peppermint, Spearmint

Still feeling those squats you did last week? Your sore muscles will thank you for adding **Nature's Ultra CBD Muscle Rub** to your regiment. CBD's anti-inflammatory properties mix with the soothing power of essential oils for your maximum relief.

- **Directions:** Apply to clean skin and massage well. Do not apply to the face, or broken and sensitive skin.
- **Ingredients:** Camellia Sinensis (Camellia) Leaf Oil, Cera Alba (Beeswax), Butyrospermum Parkii (Shea Butter), Carthamus Tinctorius (Safflower), Menthol, Squalane, Simmondsia Chinensis (Jojoba) Seed Oil, and more
- **Essential Oils:** Cinnamon Bark, Tea Tree, Lemon, Peppermint, Clove, Wintergreen, Helichrysum

Smart Spectrum™ CBD Oil Base puts you in control. Mix in your choice of essential oils to build a unique system that works for what you need, when you need it.
Available Bundles: Chill - 5ML Lavender, Pep - 5ML Peppermint

- **Directions:** Add one full dropper of plain base to your hand. Add in 2-3 drops of your favorite essential oils and apply to needed area.
- **Ingredients:** Caprylic/capric triglyceride (MCT coconut oil), Cannabidiol (CBD - 0.0 percent THC)

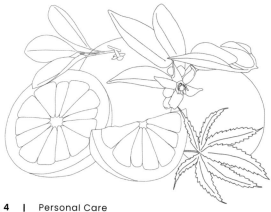

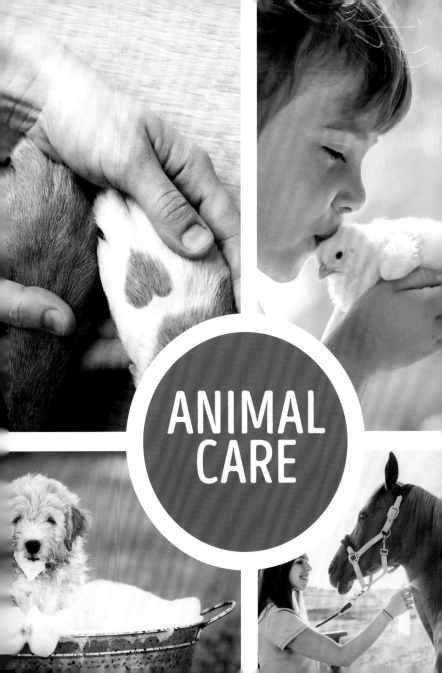

ANIMAL
CARE

ANIMAL CARE

Our furry friends benefit from oils just as much as we do! Just like with humans, essential oils are a great way to find relief for your beloved pets.

QUICK TIPS

Apply to yourself first.
- Before using essential oils on your animals, wear the oils while you spend time with them or diffuse them in common areas. This helps them adjust to the aroma and makes them less weary when applied to them.

Start slow and increase as you go!
- Animals tend to have stronger senses, especially smell, and can have different reactions to oils. A good rule of thumb is to start with 1-2 drops, get the animal used to the aroma, make sure they are comfortable and safe, and then increase if needed!

Size matters...
- This may seem self-explanatory, but we're going to say it anyway. You will not need the same amount of oils for your tiny puppy as you will for your horse! Same goes for dilution. Where you may be able to apply oils directly to larger animals, small animals may need a carrier oil or water to lower the effects.

Not all animals are alike.
- Animals are unique, just like humans. What works for your cat may not work for your dog, or even for another cat. Do not assume that because it worked on one animal it will work on all.

Take notes of what works.
- As great as it would be, our animals can't verbally share with us their experience. It's up to you to take note of changes–good and bad–and record them for future use. If you find a helpful combination and dosage, write it down so you can refer back to it later.

ANIMAL AILMENTS

Anxiety: Rub 2-3 drops of essential oil between your hands and apply it on the edge of the ears, between toes, on inner thighs, or under their front legs.
- **Recommended Oils:** Lavender, Peace & Calming, Roman Chamomile

Arthritis: Combine with carrier oil and massage onto sore joints or areas of arthritis or dysplasia. Can be applied on the inside of ear tips as well.
- **Recommended Oils:** Cool Azul Blend, OrthoEase Massage Oil, PanAway

Odor: Help your pet stay fresh by adding 1-2 drops into plain, animal friendly shampoo or combine in a spray bottle with water and mist over pet. Avoid contact with eyes.
- **Recommended Oils:** Roman Chamomile, Geranium, Lavender, Orange, Eucalyptus Radiata

Bug Repellent: Add a 1-2 drops to plain, animal friendly shampoo, apply to fabric collar, or dilute and apply 1-2 drops to the neck, back chest, legs, and tail area.
- **Recommended Oils:** Citronella, Lemon, Clary Sage, Peppermint, Lemongrass

Hyperactivity: Use aromatically by diffusing and/or rubbing together in palms and allowing them to sniff, or apply 2-3 diluted drops to the edge of your pets' ears, between toes, inner thighs, or under their front legs.
- **Recommended Oils:** Lavender, Roman Chamomile, Marjoram, Bergamot, Valerian, Peace & Calming

Motion Sickness: Combine with $\frac{1}{2}$ oz carrier oil and apply to the inside tip of the ears, under front legs, and onto belly or diffuse.
- **Recommended Oils:** Ginger, Peppermint, DiGize

Congestion: Massage several drops into neck and chest, diffuse, or add a few drops onto bedding/toys.
- **Recommended Oils:** Eucalyptus, Myrrh

Tick Repellent: Apply a few drops to the neck, back, chest, legs, and tail or add to plain, animal safe shampoo.
- **Recommended Oils:** Geranium, Bay, Lavender

Scrape Care: Combine with carrier oil and gently apply to effected area.
- **Recommended Oils:** Lavender, Helichrysum, Marjoram

ANIMAL SCENTS®

Animal Scents® Infect Away™ essential oil blend helps clean wounds and soothe irritation when your furry friend has a scrape or scratch.
- **Directions:** Carefully apply according to the size and species of the animal. Additional dilution is recommended for smaller species.
- **Ingredients:** Caprylic/Capric Glycerides
- **Essential Oils:** Myrrh, Patchouli, Dorado Azul, Palo Santo, Oregano, Ocotea

After a long outdoor adventure, park playdate, or even just messing around the house, your pet's skin may need some attention. **Animal Scents® Mendwell™** is the perfect blend to moisturize and take care of minor irritations like dryness, scratches, and scrapes.

- **Directions:** Apply 1-2 drops topically according to the size and species of animal.
- **Ingredients:** Caprylic/Capric Glycerides
- **Essential Oils:** Geranium, Lavender, Hyssop, Myrrh, Frankincense

When tummy troubles arise, reach for **Animal Scents® ParaGize™**. This specially formulated blend can be applied directly on the stomach to relieve discomfort and aid in digestion.

- **Directions:** Apply 1-2 drops to the stomach area and gently massage.
- **Essential Oils:** Ginger, Anise, Peppermint, Cumin, Spearmint, Rosemary, Juniper, Fennel, Lemongrass, Patchouli

Animal Scents® Ointment is a rich moisturizing salve that can help hydrate and soften paw pads, noses, and dry skin areas. And because it is made with 100 percent pure, natural ingredients, you don't have to worry about them licking or getting curious.

- **Directions:** Clean area and apply as needed.
- **Ingredients:** Prunus Armeniaca (Apricot) Kernel Oil, Helianthis Annuus (Sunflower) Seed Oil, Mangifera Indica (Mango) Seed Butter, and more
- **Essential Oils:** Palmarosa, Carrot Seed, Geranium, Patchouli, Coriander, Grape, Balsam, Myrrh, Tea Tree (Melaleuca Alternifolia), Bergamot, Ylang Ylang

We love our pets... but they can get gross! Clean them up with **Animal Scents® Toxin Free Shampoo**. Tough on dirt and germs, but gentle on skin, this toxin-free shampoo helps your pet get the best clean, soft, moisturized, healthy-looking coat around!

- **Directions:** Gently massage through a pet's wet coat. Lather. Rinse thoroughly. Repeat if necessary.
- **Ingredients:** Decyl Glucoside, Coco-Betaine, Lauryl Glucoside, Coco-Glucoside, Glycerin, Glyceryl Oleate, Citric Acid, Xanthan Gum, and more
- **Essential Oils:** Lavandin, Lemon, Geranium, Citronella, Northern Lights Black Spruce, Vetiver

Provide a nice, calming environment for your animals with **Animal Scents® T-Away™**. Perfect for time home alone, drives in the car, or any other stressful experience, this soothing blend helps support your furry friends and promote more joy and balance.

- **Directions:** Apply 1 drop behind each ear to calm your pet.
- **Ingredients:** Caprylic/Capric Glycerides
- **Essential Oils:** Tangerine, Lavender, Royal Hawaiian Sandalwood, German Chamomile, Frankincense, Valerian, Ylang Ylang, Black Spruce, Geranium, Davana, Orange, Rue, Lime, Patchouli, Coriander, Blue Tansy, Bergamot, Rose, Lemon, Jasmine, Roman Chamomile, Palmarosa

OTHER OILS FOR ANIMALS & AILMENTS

Thieves-
Bacterial/Inflammation/Infection/Burns/Splinters: Dab 1-2 drops gently to affected area.

Frankincense-
Seizures/Injuries: Tap 1-4 drops into your palm, rub palms together, and pet animal on the spine, neck and chest.

Lavender-
Tissue regeneration, infection, and calming. Effective against ringworm. Use 1-4 drops topically on area.

DiGize-
Motion Sickness/Vomiting/Stomach Pain: Tap 1-4 drops on your palm, rub palms together and pet animal on the spine, neck, chest, and stomach.

Purification-
Insect Bites/Stings/Nettle/Poison Ivy and Oak/Coughing: Tap 1-2 drops on your palm and dab gently to affected area.

Cistus-
Scrapes: Place 1-4 drops directly to the affected area, then pet animal gently on the spine, neck, and chest.

Raven-
Respiratory Infections/Breathing Difficulties: Tap 1-4 drops into your palm, rub palms together and pet animal on the spine, neck, and chest.

Peppermint-
Vomiting/Heat Stroke/Lethargy: Tap 1-4 drops into your palm, rub palms together and pet animal on the spine, neck, and chest.

PanAway-
Inflammation/Ear Mites/Ear Infections/Ticks: Dilute with carrier oil and apply directly to affected area. Avoid open, raw tissue.

OrthoEase Massage Oil-
Chronic Pain/Arthritis: Squirt 1 pump on your palm, rub palms together, and gently pet the animal on affected area(s). Avoid open wounds.

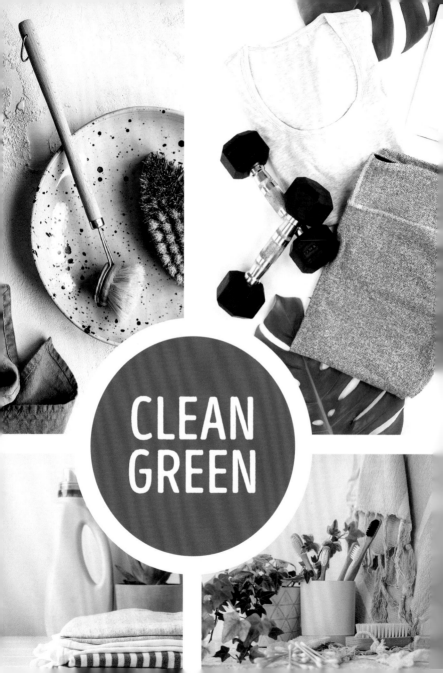

CLEAN GREEN

CLEAN GREEN

Formaldehyde... Perchloroethylene... Butoxyethanol... No thank you! We all want a clean home, but so many of today's cleaning agents are filled with harsh chemicals that can do more harm than good. Luckily, there are safe alternatives that keep your home clean AND toxin free!

Free from harsh chemicals, **Thieves® Household Cleaner** is your "can do" versatile cleaner that harnesses powerful antibacterial and purifying essential oils to achieve the clean you need with ingredients you can trust.

- **Directions:** Most cleaning applications: 1 capful of Thieves Household Cleaner and 2 cups of water. Light degreasing: 1 capful of Thieves Household Cleaner and 4 cups of water.
- **Ingredients:** Water, Alkyl Polyglucoside, Sodium 2-Methyl Sulfolaurate, Tetrasodium Glutamate Diacetate, Disodium 2-Sulfolaurate
- **Essential Oils:** Clove, Lemon, Cinnamon, Rosemary, Eucalyptus Radiata

Laundry goals start with **Thieves® Laundry Soap**. Potent, plant-based, and ultra-concentrated with pure essential oils, this natural cleanser uses powerful enzymes to effectively clean your clothes and leave them refreshed with a light citrus scent.

- **Directions:** Follow the instructions found on the garment's care label. Add clothes. Start machine and add the proper amount of soap for load size. Standard load: $\frac{1}{2}$ cap for conventional washers, $\frac{1}{4}$ cap for HE washers. Use more, as needed, for large or heavily soiled loads.
- **Ingredients:** Water, Decyl Glucoside, Sodium Oleate, Glycerin, Caprylyl Glucoside, Lauryl Glucoside, Sodium Chloride, Sodium Gluconate, Carboxymethyl Cellulose, and more
- **Essential Oils:** Lemon, Bergamot, Jade Lemon, Clove, Cinnamon, Eucalyptus Radiata, Rosemary

Need a quick clean? **Thieves® Wipes** are a convenient, natural way to purify your hard surfaces. A simple rub disinfects the desired area, picking up any remains as you wipe, and leave nothing but the signature Thieves scent behind.

- **Directions:** Wipe desired area thoroughly.
- **Ingredients:** Alcohol, Water, Sunflower Lecithin, Quillaja Saponaria Extract
- **Essential Oils:** Clove, Lemon, Cinnamon Bark, Eucalyptus Radiata, Rosemary

Keep your produce fresher and longer with **Thieves® Fruit & Veggie Soak.** Adding this all-natural formula to your washing routine safely washes away dirt, pesticides, and other contaminants, so you can enjoy your fruits and vegetables with peace of mind.

- **Directions:** 1 ounce (2 tablespoons) for every gallon of water. Completely cover produce and soak for 1-2 minutes. Rinse with clean water.
- **Ingredients:** Water, Decyl Glucoside, Glycerin, Citric Acid, Sodium Citrate
- **Essential Oils:** Tarragon, Ginger, Peppermint, Juniper, Fennel, Lemongrass, Clove, Rosemary, Citronella, Anise, Lemon, Patchouli, Cinnamon, Tea Tree (Melaleuca Alternifolia), Lavandin, Eucalyptus Radiata, Myrtle

Pump it up! Thieves® Foaming Hand Soap combines effective, plant-derived ingredients and powerful moisturizers to thoroughly clean hands without drying your skin.

- **Directions:** Lather and rub hands together for 20 seconds then rinse completely with warm water.
- **Ingredients:** Water, Decyl Glucoside, Alcohol Denat., Cetyl Hydroxyethyl Cellulose, Glycerin, Sodium Hydroxide, Camellia Sinensis Leaf Extract, Ginkgo Biloba Leaf Extract, Aloe Barbadensis Leaf Juice Powder, Tocopherol, Helianthus Annuus (Sunflower) Seed Oil, Citric Acid
- **Essential Oils:** Clove, Orange, Lemon, Cinnamon Bark, Eucalyptus Radiata, Rosemary

Sparkling clean dishes start with **Thieves® Automatic Dishwasher Powder.** Natural enzymes, earth-derived botanicals, and Young Living's signature Thieves premium essential oil blend combine to effectively sanitize dishes with every wash.

- **Directions:** Place 1 scoop of Thieves Automatic Dishwasher Powder in the dishwasher dispenser. Use 2 scoops for heavy loads or with hard water. For an extra boost, add a small amount of citric acid.
- **Ingredients:** Sodium Carbonate, Sodium Citrate Dihydrate, Sodium Percarbonate, Sodium Silicate, Sapindus Mukorossi (Soapberry) Fruit Extract, Tapioca Maltodextrin, Silica, Protease, Helianthus Annuus (Sunflower) Oil, Amylase
- **Essential Oils:** Orange, Lemongrass, Clove, Lemon, Cinnamon Bark, Rosemary, Eucalyptus Radiata

Food stuck on your plate? Dish please... **Thieves® Dish Soap** is tough on grease and grime, gentle on hands, and has a fresh, citrus scent—all powered by natural cleansing agents and premium essential oils.

- **Directions:** Dispense a small amount of soap with warm running water. Add additional soap as needed.
- **Ingredients:** Water, Decyl Glucoside, Sodium Lauroyl Lactylate, Lauryl Glucoside, Caprylyl Glucoside
- **Essential Oils:** Lemon, Bergamot, Jade Lemon, Clove, Cinnamon Bark, Eucalyptus Radiata, Rosemary

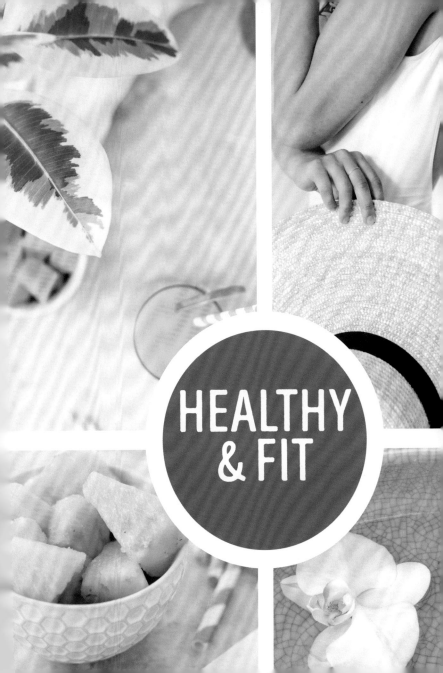

HEALTHY
& FIT

HEALTHY & FIT

NINGXIA® WOLFBERRY

Get up and get going with **NingXia Nitro™**! This all-natural, power packed paste is a great way to increase cognitive alertness, enhance mental fitness, promote energy, and support overall performance, all while avoiding the typical caffeine crash.

- **Directions:** Consume NingXia Nitro® directly from the tube or mix with 1 oz. of NingXia Red® or 4 oz. of water to enhance physical performance, clear the mind, or anytime you need a pick-me-up. Best served chilled. Shake well before use.
- **Ingredients:** D-Ribose, Green tea extract, Mulberry leaf extract, Korean ginseng extract, Proprietary Nitro Alert™ oil blend, Coconut nectar, and more
- **Essential Oils:** Vanilla, Spearmint, Peppermint, Nutmeg, Black Pepper

NingXia Red® is a more than just a delicious drink. Ningxia wolfberries have long been treasured in the natural health community. Their phytochemical profile is legendary: amazing polysaccharides, calcium, 18 amino acids, 21 trace minerals, beta-carotene, vitamins B1, B2, B6, and E, along with polyphenols. Packed with all these powerful antioxidants, NingXia is here to help you feel your very best!

- **Directions:** Drink 1-2 fl. oz., 2 times daily. Combine with NingXia Nitro for a nourishing drink that also supports cognitive wellness. Best served chilled. Shake well before use. Refrigerate after opening and consume within 30 days.
- **Ingredients:** Ningxia Wolfberry Puree (Lycium barbarum), Blueberry Juice Concentrate (Vaccinium corymbosum), and more
- **Essential Oils:** Grape, Orange, Yuzu, Lemon, Tangerine

Add some extra pep to you day. **NingXia Zyng™** is a light, sparkling beverage that delivers a splash of hydrating energy. It is fueled by a proprietary blend of pure Black Pepper and Lime essential oils, wolfberry puree, and white tea extract, combined with vitamins to create a unique, delicious, and refreshing beverage.

- **Directions:** Drink one can as desired. Lightly invert can before opening.
- **Ingredients:** Carbonated water, Evaporated cane sugar, Pear juice concentrate, Wolfberry (Lycium barbarum) puree, Citric acid, Blackberry juice concentrate, Natural flavor, White tea leaf extract, Stevia rebaudiana leaf extract, D-calcium pantothenate, Niacinamide, D-alpha-tocopherol acetate, Pyridoxine hydrochloride, Retinyl palmitate.
- **Essential Oils:** Black Pepper, Lime

Young Living's **Ningxia organic Dried Wolfberries** are a great sweet, organic snack from nature that's easy to make a part of your daily diet.

- **Directions:** Store in a cool, dark place. Enjoy ½ oz. (approx. 1 Tbsp.) as desired – eat raw, add to oatmeal and pancakes, mix in salads, make jams and jellies, steep into tea, and more.
- **Ingredients:** Whole Dried Organic Ningxia Wolfberries

SUPPLEMENTS

Help bring some extra balance to your life with the **Balance Complete**™ super-food meal replacement. High in fiber and protein, it is an effective approach to weight-loss goals and helps support a healthy immune system, muscle growth and recovery, and cleansing of the digestive system.

- **Directions:** Add two scoops of Balance Complete to 8-10 ounces of cold water or milk of your choice. Shake, stir or blend until smooth
- **Ingredients:** Proprietary V-Fiber™ Blend, Whey Protein Concentrate, Nonfat Dry Milk, Mediumchain Triglycerides, Magnesium Oxide, Aloe Vera Leaf, Mixed Tocopherols, and more
- **Essential Oils:** Orange

Keep your mind sharp and your heart healthy with the **MindWise**™ **Dietary Supplement.** Regular usage supports healthy cardiovascular and cognitive health with CoQ10, ALCR, and GPC ingredients, plus fruit juices and extracts, turmeric, and premium essential oils.

- **Directions:** Take 2 tablespoons (6 teaspoons) once daily for the first 7-10 days. After first week, take 1 tablespoon (3 teaspoons) once daily or as needed.
- **Ingredients:** Proprietary Mindwise Memory Blend, Proprietary MindWise Oil Blend, Water, Pomegranate (Punica granatum) juice concentrate, and more
- **Essential Oils:** Lemon, Peppermint, Fennel, Lime

Your heart is a delicate thing! Treat it right with **CardioGize**™ **Herbal Supplement.** This formula blends vital CoQ10, selenium, and vitamin K2 with supportive herbals to fill in any gaps that your heart may need.

- **Directions:** Take 2 capsules daily. Store in a cool, dark place.
- **Ingredients:** Hypromellose, Water, Silica, Proprietary Healthy Heart Blend
- **Essential Oils:** Angelica, Cardamom, Cypress, Lavender, Helichrysum, Rosemary, Cinnamon Bark

Many foods naturally contain enzymes that help break down and process nutrients. However, these enzymes can be destroyed in the cooking process. **Essentialzyme™** is specially formulated to support and balance digestive health and to stimulate overall enzyme activity to combat the modern diet.

- **Directions:** Take 1 dual time-release caplet 1 hour before your largest meal of the day for best results.
- **Ingredients:** Proprietary Blend (Light): Pancrealipase, Pancreatin, Trypsin Proprietary Blend (Dark): Betaine HCl, Bromelain, Thyme (Thymus Vulgaris) Leaf Powder, Carrot (Daucus Carota) Root Powder, and more
- **Essential Oils:** Anise, Fennel, Peppermint, Tarragon, Clove

Get those greens! **MultiGreens™ Herbal Supplement** is a nutritious chlorophyll and essential oil capsule designed to boost vitality by working with the glandular, nervous, and circulatory systems.

- **Directions:** Take 3 capsules, 2 times daily.
- **Ingredients:** Bee Pollen, Barley Grass Juice Concentrate, Spirulina, Choline, Eleuthero Root, Alfalfa Stem/Leaf Extract, Kelp Whole Thallus, and more
- **Essential Oils:** Rosemary, Lemon, Lemongrass, Melissa

Feeling sluggish? It might be time for a detox! While that word may sound intimidating, **Detoxzyme®** makes it easy. This dietary supplement combines a myriad of powerful enzymes that complete digestion, help detoxify, and promote cleansing in harmony with your body's natural abilities.

- **Directions:** Take 2 capsules, three times daily, between meals or as needed. This product may be used in conjunction with a cleansing or detoxifying program. For the relief of occasional symptoms such as fullness, pressure, bloating, gas, pain, and/or minor cramping that may occur after eating.
- **Ingredients:** Amylase, Cumin (Cuminum Cyminum) Seed Powder, Invertase, Protease 4.5, Glucoamylase, Bromelain, Phytase, and more
- **Essential Oils:** Cumin, Anise, Fennel

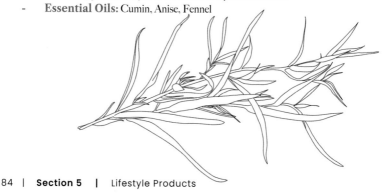

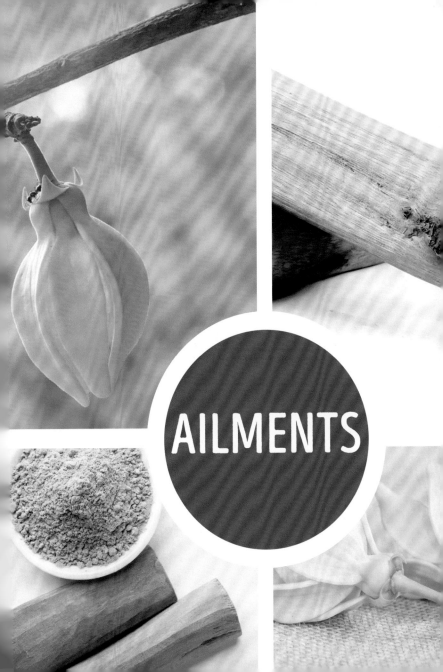

AILMENTS

COMMON AILMENTS

ACNE
- **Products:** Melrose™, Purification®, Geranium, Vetiver, Sandalwood, Patchouli, Lavender, German or Roman Chamomile, Melaleuca Quinquenervia, ART® Skin Care System, Mineral Essence™, Detoxzyme
- **Usage:** Apply 3-5 drops neat or diluted 50/50 on affected area, 2-4 times daily Alternate oils, as desired.

ARTHRITIS/JOINT PAIN
- **Products:** PanAway®, Relieve It™, Aroma Siez™, Deep Relief Roll-on, Idaho Balsam Fir, Frankincense, Palo Santo, ICP™, JuvaPower™, Sulfurzyme™, BLM™, Detoxzyme
- **Usage:** Apply 3-5 drops neat or diluted 50/50 on affected area, 2-4 times daily. Alternate oils as desired.

ATHLETE'S FOOT/RINGWORM
- **Products:** Melrose™, Thieves®, Purification®, Patchouli, Melaleuca, (M. Alternifolia), Blue Cypress, Lavender, Peppermint, Thyme, Melissa
- **Usage:** Apply 3-5 drops neat or diluted 50/50 on affected area, 2-4 times daily. Alternate oils, as desired.

ATTENTION DEFICIT (ADD and ADHD)
- **Products:** Brain Power™, Peace & Calming®, Clarity™, Common Sense™, RutaVaLa™ (oil or roll-on), Vetiver, Lavender, Cedarwood, Peppermint, Frankincense
- **Usage:** Diffuse 15 minutes, 4-8 times daily. Massage 3-5 drops on brain stem, back of the neck, and temples.

BACKACHE/LUMBAGO
- **Products:** Aroma Siez™, PanAway®, Relieve It™, Deep Relief Roll-On, Lavender, Idaho Balsam Fir, Wintergreen, Marjoram, Copaiba, Peppermint
- **Usage:** Apply 3-5 drops neat or diluted 50/50 on affected area, 2-4 times daily. Alternate oils, as desired.

BLISTERS/BOILS
- **Products:** LavaDerm Cooling Mist, Purification®, Melrose™, Melaleuca (M. Alternifolia), Myrrh, Lavender, Rose Ointment, Spikenard
- **Usage:** Apply 3-5 drops neat or diluted 50/50 on affected area, every 2-3 hours.
- Alternate oils, as desired.

BRUISED MUSCLES
- **Products:** German Chamomile, Spikenard, Cistus, Marjoram, Wintergreen, Helichrysum, Cypress, PanAway®, Deep Relief Roll-On, Relieve It™
- **Usage:** Apply 3-5 drops neat or diluted 50/50 on affected area, 4-6 times daily.

BUG/INSECT/SPIDER BITES, BEE STINGS, ETC.
- **Products:** Idaho Tansy, Palo Santo, Thieves®, Purification®, Peppermint, Eucalyptus Blue, Dorado Azul, Citronella, Lemongrass, Melrose™, Lavender
- **Usage:** Mix Idaho Tansy and Palo Santo and spray undiluted or mixed with 1/2 cup of water on skin, clothing and bedding. Add 5-10 drops of other oils. Spray Thieves® or Purification® neat or diluted in water. Apply 1-2 drops of chosen oil on area. Your choice of combination.

BURNS/SUNBURNS
- **Products:** LavaDerm, Cooling Mist, Spikenard, Lavender, Idaho Balsam Fir, Helichrysum, Valor®, Gentle Baby™, Australian Blue™, Melrose™
- **Usage:** Spray as often as needed. Add 3-5 drops of other oil(s) to LavaDerm or other spray mixture as desired, and spray or apply 3-5 drops neat or diluted 50/50 on affected area every hour, or as needed.

CIRCULATION PROBLEMS (BLOOD)
- **Products:** Helichrysum, Cypress, Tangerine, Idaho Balsam Fir, En-R-Gee™, Aroma Life™, EndoFlex™, Valor® (oil or roll-on), NingXia Red®
- **Usage:** Apply 2-4 drops neat or diluted 50/50 on desired areas. Have a body massage weekly.

COLD SORES (HERPES SIMPLEX TYPE 1)
- **Products:** Melrose™, Purification®, Melissa, Thieves®, Myrrh, Melaleuca (M. Alternifolia), Lavender, Sandalwood, Vetiver, Patchouli, Ravintsara
- **Usage:** Apply 1 drop of chosen oil neat or directly on cold sore every 1-2 hours.

COLDS/FLU/INFLUENZA
- **Products:** Raven™, ImmuPower™, Thieves®, DiGize™, Exodus II™, R.C.™, Mountain Savory, Oregano, Eucalyptus Blue, Peppermint, Clove, Dorado Azul, Inner Defense, Thieves® Mouthwash, Detoxzyme
- **Usage:** Diffuse 30-45 minutes. Inhale directly, 2-4 times daily. Apply 3-4 drops neat or diluted on the throat, chest, and back.

CUTS/SCRAPES/WOUNDS
- **Products:** Melrose™, Aroma Life™, Rosemary, Eucalyptus (E. Globulus), Dorado Azul, Thyme, Lavender, Melaleuca (M. Alternifolia), Frankincense, Helichrysum
- **Usage:** Apply 3-5 drops neat or diluted 50/50 on affected area, 2-4 times daily. Alternate oils to determine best effect.

DANDRUFF
- **Products:** Cedar Wood, Rosemary, Melrose™, Thieves®, Citrus Fresh™, Melaleuca (M. Alternifolia), Eucalyptus Blue, Lavender, Lavender Mint Shampoo
- **Usage:** Massage vigorously 1 tsp of desired oil neat or diluted 50/50 into scalp for 2-3 minutes; leave for 15 minutes and then shampoo.

DEPRESSION
- **Products:** RutaVaLa™ (oil or roll-on), Hope™, The Gift™, Frankincense, Live with Passion™, Valor® (oil or roll-on), Melissa, Inspiration™, Jasmine, Rose, Mineral Essence, Thyromin, Balance Complete™
- **Usage:** Gently massage 2-3 drops on rim of ears. Diffuse 20-30 minutes, 3-4 times daily or as desired. Inhale directly, 4-6 times daily.

DIZZINESS/FAINTING
- **Products:** Clarity™, Awaken™, Brain Power™, Common Sense™, Highest Potential™, Grounding™, Ocotea, Eucalyptus Blue, Peppermint, NingXia Red®, MultiGreens
- **Usage:** Apply 1-2 drops neat to the crown, brainstem, and forehead, as needed. Diffuse 30-45 minutes, 4-5 times daily. Inhale directly throughout the day, as needed, breathing slowly and deeply.

ECZEMA/DERMATITIS/SKIN DISORDERS
- **Products:** Juva Cleanse®, Purification®, Melrose™, Australian Blue™, Cistus, Blue Cypress, Roman Chamomile, Lavender, German Chamomile, Myrrh, Patchouli
- **Usage:** Apply 4-5 drops neat or diluted 50/50 on affected area, as needed.

EMOTIONAL TRAUMA
- **Products:** Hope™, The Gift™, RutaVaLa™ (oil or roll-on), Trauma Life, Peace & Calming®, Joy™, Inspiration™, Sacred Frankincense™, Valerian, Lavender, Rose, Galbanum
- **Usage:** Diffuse 30-40 minutes, 4-5 times daily, or as desired. Inhale directly throughout the day, as needed. Apply 1-2 drops neat to the crown, brainstem, and forehead, as needed.

FEVER
- **Products:** Peppermint, Eucalyptus Blue, ImmuPower™, Melrose™, Palo Santo, Spearmint, Orange, Idaho Balsam Fir, Myrrh, M-Grain™, Dorado Azul
- **Usage:** Apply 2-3 drops of neat or diluted 50/50 to forehead, temples, and back of neck.

FRIGIDITY/SEXUAL DYSFUNCTION

- **Products:** SclarEssence™, Sensation™, Lady Sclareol™, Mister™, Into the Future™, Motivation™, Valor®, Joy™, Ylang Ylang, Jasmine
- **Usage:** Inhale directly, as desired. Apply 1-2 drops neat or diluted 50/50 on neck, shoulders, and lower abdomen, 1-3 times daily.

GUM DISEASE

- **Products:** Thieves®, Melrose™, PanAway®, Thieves® Dentarome Toothpaste, Thieves® Mouthwash, Clove, Peppermint, Melaleuca (M. Alternifolia), Thyme
- **Usage:** Gargle with chosen oil, as needed.

HALITOSIS/BAD BREATH

- **Products:** Thieves®, Purification®, DiGize™, Peppermint, Lemon, Spearmint, Cassia, Ocotea, Essentialzyme, Detoxzyme, Digest & Cleanse, Life 9™
- **Usage:** Gargle, 2-4 times daily, as needed. Put 1-2 drops on tongue, as desired.

HEADACHE

- **Products:** M-Grain™, PanAway®, Brain Power™, Clarity™, Deep Relief Roll-On, Stress Away™ Roll-On, Dorado Azul, Eucalyptus Blue, Roman Chamomile, NingXia Red®, ComforTone, Essentialzyme
- **Usage:** Apply 1-3 drops neat or diluted 50/50 on back of neck, behind ears, on temples, on forehead, and under nose. Diffuse 15-30 minutes, 3-5 times daily. Inhale directly, 3-8 times daily, as needed.

HIGH BLOOD PRESSURE (HYPERTENSION)

- **Products:** Cypress, Helichrysum, Marjoram, Aroma Life™, Peace & Calming®, Ocotea, Lavender, Ylang Ylang, RutaVaLa™ (oil or roll-on) Essentialzyme, OmegaGize3®, Mineral Essence, Citrus Fresh™
- **Usage:** Dilute, body massage daily. Diffuse daily.

HIVES

- **Products:** Myrrh, German Chamomile, Ravintsara, Lavender, RutaVaLa™ (oil or roll-on) Stress Away™ Roll-On, Peace & Calming®
- **Usage:** Apply 2-4 drops neat or diluted 50/50 on location, as needed.

INSOMNIA

- **Products:** RutaVaLa™ (oil or roll-on), Peace & Calming®, SleepEssence, Valor® (oil or roll-on), Stress Away™ Roll-On, Lavender, Cedar Wood, Valerian
- **Usage:** Apply neat 1-3 drops to shoulders, stomach, and on bottoms of feet. Diffuse 30 minutes at bedtime.

LIVER CLEANSING

- **Products:** JuvaFlex™, Ledum, Celery Seed, Lemon, Orange, Rosemary, Juva Cleanse®, Release™, Detoxzyme, JuvaPower, German Chamomile, ComforTone
- **Usage:** Place warm compress over the liver 1 time daily for 15-30 minutes.

MUSCLE CRAMPS/SPASMS

- **Products:** PanAway®, Relieve It™, Aroma Siez™, Rosemary, Marjoram, Vetiver, Deep Relief Roll-On, Ortho Ease and Ortho Sport Massage Oils, MegaCal, Mineral Essence
- **Usage:** Massage 2-4 drops neat or diluted 50/50 on cramped muscle, 3 times daily. It may help to alternate cold and hot packs on affected muscle.

NAUSEA/MOTION SICKNESS

- **Products:** DiGize™, Juva Cleanse®, GLF™, Ginger, Nutmeg, Ocotea, Peppermint, AlkaLime, Detoxzyme, Essentialzyme, Spearmint, Valor® (oil or roll-on), Patchouli
- **Usage:** Massage 1-3 drops neat or diluted 50/50 behind each ear and over naval, 2-3 times hourly. Put 1 drop on tongue, 1-3 times daily, or as needed. Inhale directly, 4-6 times hourly, as desired.

PAIN

- **Products:** PanAway®, Deep Relief Roll-On, Relieve It™, Aroma Siez™, Peppermint, Dorado Azul, Palo Santo, Idaho Balsam Fir, Valerian, Ortho Sport Massage Oil
- **Usage:** Apply 2-4 drops neat or diluted 50/50 on location, as needed.

PARASITES

- **Products:** ParaFree, Thieves®, DiGize™, Juva Cleanse®, Lemongrass, Tarragon, Anise, Basil, ICP, ComforTone, Detoxzyme, Life 6™
- **Usage:** Place a warm compress over intestinal area, 2 times weekly.

PMS/MENSTRUAL AND HORMONE CONDITIONS

- **Products:** SclarEssence™, Dragon Time™, EndoFlex™, Lady Sclareol™, Rose, Progessence Plus Serum (1-2 drops on neck or as directed), Prenolone Plus Body Cream, Clary Sage, Fennel, Ylang Ylang
- **Usage:** Apply 4-6 drops neat or diluted 50/50 on the forehead, crown of head, soles of feet, lower abdomen, and lower back, 1-3 times daily. Inhale directly throughout the day, as desired.

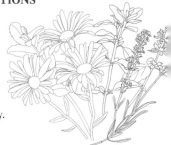

PNEUMONIA/BRONCHITIS
- **Products:** Raven™, Melrose™, R.C.™, Thieves®, Exodus II™, Thyme, Ravintsara, Eucalyptus (E. Radiata), Oregano, Inner Defense™, Breathe Again™ Roll-On, Super C (or chewable), Mountain Savory
- **Usage:** Diffuse different oils for 15-30 minutes, 3-8 times daily. Inhale directly, 5-10 times daily, as needed, alternating oils. Apply 2-6 drops neat or diluted 50/50 over neck, back, and chest as needed.

RESTLESS LEG SYNDROME
- **Products:** Aroma Siez™, Peace & Calming®, RutaVaLa™ (oil or roll-on), Stress Away™ Roll-On, Mineral Essence, Basil, Marjoram, Lavender, Cypress, Roman Chamomile, Valerian
- **Usage:** Massage 6-8 drops of oil neat or diluted 50/50 on the leg, 3-4 times daily, as needed. Apply 3-4 drops neat to the Vita Flex points on the feet before retiring.

SHINGLES
- **Products:** Blue Cypress, Australian Blue™, Exodus II™, Thieves®, Elemi, Idaho Tansy, Melaleuca (M. Alternifolia), Lavender, Super Cal, Sulfurzyme, Ravintsara, Melaleuca Quinquenervia
- **Usage:** Apply 6-10 drops neat or diluted 50/50 on affected areas, back of neck, and down the spine, 1-3 times daily.

SINUS CONGESTION/INFECTION
- **Products:** DiGize™, Raven™, Thieves®, Exodus II™, Breathe Again™ Roll-On, Peppermint, Eucalyptus Blue, Palo Santo, Eucalyptus (E. Radiata), Ravintsara, R.C.™
- **Usage:** Inhale directly, 3-8 times daily, as needed. Put 1-2 drops of oil in water and gargle, 3-6 times daily. Massage 1-3 drops neat or diluted 50/50 on forehead, nose, cheeks, lower throat, chest, and upper back.

SORE MUSCLES
- **Products:** PanAway®, Deep Relief Roll-On, Aroma Siez™, Relieve It™, Dorado Azul, Copaiba, Wintergreen, Marjoram, Peppermint, MegaCal, Mineral Essence, Ortho Ease and Ortho Sport Massage Oils
- **Usage:** Massage sore muscles, oil neat or diluted 50/50. Apply a warm compress on location.

SORE THROAT/COUGH
- **Products:** Thieves®, Thieves® Lozenges, Thieves® Spray, Eucalyptus (E. Radiata), Lemon, Peppermint, Super C (or chewable), Exodus II™, Ocotea, Eucalyptus Blue, Dorado Azul, R.C.™
- **Usage:** Put 1 drop on the tongue, 2-6 times daily. Gargle, 4-8 times daily. Inhale directly, 3-6 times daily. Apply 1-3 drops neat or diluted 50/50 on throat, chest, and back of neck, 2-4 times daily.

SPRAIN/MUSCLE INFLAMMATION
- **Products:** PanAway®, Aroma Siez™, Deep Relief Roll-On, Relieve It™, Wintergreen, Idaho Balsam Fir, Helichrysum, Mineral Essence, Peppermint, Lavender, BLM
- **Usage:** Apply 4-6 drops neat or diluted 50/50 on location, 3-5 times daily. Apply a cold compress on location, 2 times daily.

STREP THROAT
- **Products:** Exodus II™, Melrose™, Thieves®, Eucalyptus (E. Globulus), Inner Defense, ImmuPro, Frankincense, Super C (or chewable), Myrrh, Dorado Azul, Eucalyptus Blue
- **Usage:** Put 1 drop on the tongue, 2-6 times daily, as needed. Gargle, 4-8 times daily. Inhale, 3-6 times daily. Apply 1-3 drops neat or diluted 50/50 on throat, chest, and back of neck, 2-4 times daily.

STRESS/FATIGUE
- **Products:** RutaVaLa™ (oil or roll-on), Stress Away™ Roll-On, Peace & Calming®, Valor®, Lavender, Valerian, MultiGreens, Power Meal, NingXia Red®, Sandalwood
- **Usage:** Inhale directly as needed. Diffuse 30-45 minutes, 1-3 times daily. Apply 2-3 drops on temples, neck, and shoulders, 2 times daily or as needed.

URINARY/BLADDER INFECTION
- **Products:** K & B, ImmuPro, Myrrh, EndoFlex™, R.C.™, Melrose™, Thieves®, Spikenard, AlkaLime, Inspiration™, Rosemary, Juniper, Oregano, DiGize™
- **Usage:** Apply a warm compress for 15-20 minutes over bladder area, 1-2 times daily.

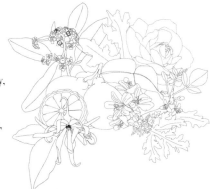

VITA FLEX LEFT FOOT

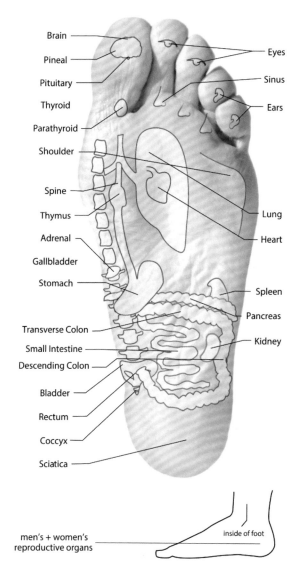

Brain
Pineal
Pituitary
Thyroid
Parathyroid
Shoulder
Spine
Thymus
Adrenal
Gallbladder
Stomach
Transverse Colon
Small Intestine
Descending Colon
Bladder
Rectum
Coccyx
Sciatica

Eyes
Sinus
Ears
Lung
Heart
Spleen
Pancreas
Kidney

men's + women's
reproductive organs

inside of foot

VITA FLEX RIGHT FOOT

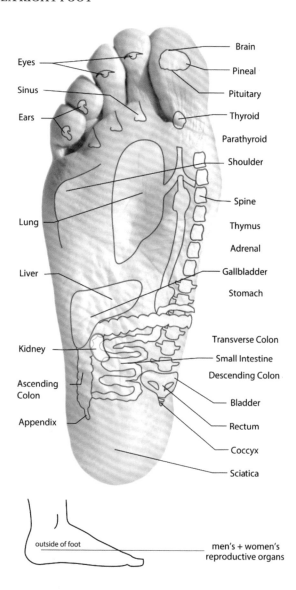

Brain

Eyes

Pineal

Sinus

Pituitary

Ears

Thyroid

Parathyroid

Shoulder

Spine

Lung

Thymus

Adrenal

Liver

Gallbladder

Stomach

Transverse Colon

Kidney

Small Intestine

Descending Colon

Ascending Colon

Bladder

Appendix

Rectum

Coccyx

Sciatica

outside of foot

men's + women's reproductive organs

VITA FLEX LEFT HAND

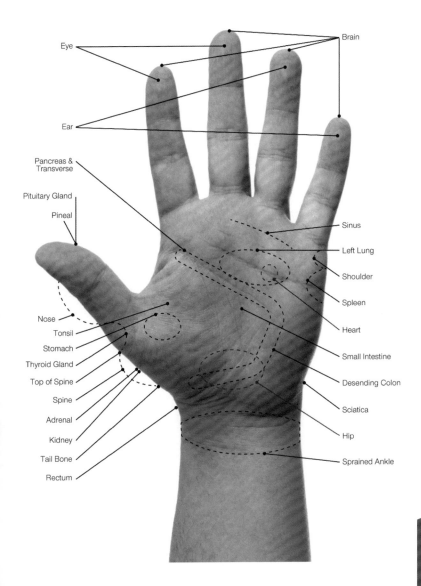

Brain

Eye

Ear

Pancreas & Transverse

Pituitary Gland

Pineal

Sinus

Left Lung

Shoulder

Spleen

Nose

Tonsil

Stomach

Thyroid Gland

Top of Spine

Spine

Adrenal

Kidney

Tail Bone

Rectum

Heart

Small Intestine

Desending Colon

Sciatica

Hip

Sprained Ankle

VITA FLEX RIGHT HAND

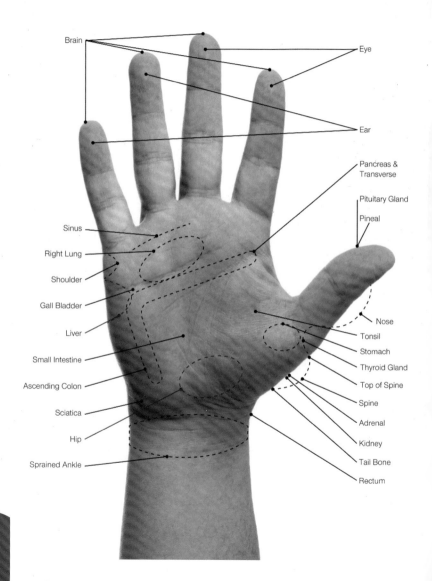